D0006413

CONQUERING
CHRONIC DISEASE
THROUGH MAHARISHI VEDIC MEDICINE

OTHER BOOKS BY DR. KUMUDA REDDY:

Forever Healthy—*Introduction to Maharishi Ayur-Veda Health Care*
by Kumuda Reddy, M.D. and Stan Kendz

For A Blissful Baby: Healthy and Happy Pregnancy
with Maharishi Vedic Medicine
by Kumuda Reddy, M.D., Linda Egenes, M.A. and
Margaret Mullins, MSN, CFNP.

All Love Flows to the Self: Eternal Stories from the Upanishads
by Kumuda Reddy, M.D., Thomas Egenes and Linda Egenes

The *Timeless Wisdom* Series of children's stories,
by Kumuda Reddy, M.D. and John Pruitt:

The Indigo Jackal
The Lion and the Hare
The Monkey and the Crocodile
The Female Mouse
The Hares and the Elephants

Samhita Productions' website: http://allhealthyfamily.com

ABOUT THE AUTHORS

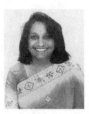

Dr. Kumuda Reddy has been practicing medicine for twenty-five years. She completed her residency and fellowship in anesthesiology at Mt. Sinai Hospital, New York. For many years, she was a faculty member and anesthesiologist at Albany Medical College. Currently she is Medical Director of the Maharishi Vedic Health Center in Bethesda, Maryland. Dr. Reddy has authored several books on Maharishi Vedic Medicine, including *Forever Healthy—Introduction to Maharishi Ayur-Veda Health Care* and *For a Blissful Baby: Healthy and Happy Pregnancy with Maharishi Vedic Medicine*, and the forthcoming *Golden Transition: Menopause Made Easy with Maharishi Vedic Medicine* and *Living Life Free from Pain: Treating Arthritis, Joint Pain, Muscle Pain and Fibromyalgia with Maharishi Vedic Medicine*. Dr. Reddy has also co-authored a book of stories from the Upanishads, entitled *All Love Flows to the Self*, and a series of children's stories called the Timeless Wisdom Series, based on traditional Indian stories that she first heard as a child on her grandmother's knee.

In addition to her life as a doctor and a writer, Dr. Reddy is a devoted wife and a mother. She lives in Bethesda with her husband Janardhan, also an M.D. and fellow expert in Maharishi Vedic Medicine, and their three children, Sundeep, Hima, and Suma.

Linda Egenes is the author of several books and has written about Maharishi Vedic Medicine for the past thirteen years. She teaches in the M.A. in Professional Writing program at Maharishi University of Management in Fairfield, Iowa, where she lives with her husband, Tom.

WNCC Library
16 NO LONGER Street
S PROPERTY OF 69361
WNCC Library

CONQUERING CHRONIC DISEASE
THROUGH MAHARISHI VEDIC MEDICINE

by
Kumuda Reddy, M.D.
with Linda Egenes, M.A.

Samhita Productions
Schenectady, New York

APR 16 2002

All illustrations courtesy of Kathryn Peckman, Jo Ann Gessner and Craig Ridgley

Published by Lantern Books
1 Union Square West, Suite 201, New York, New York 10003

©2002 by Maharishi Vedic Education Development Corporation and Kumuda Reddy, M.D.

All rights reserved. No part of this book may be reproduced, stored in a retrieval system, or transmitted in any form or by any means, electronic, mechanical, photocopying, recording, or otherwise, without prior written permission of the publisher, except by a reviewer who may quote brief passages in a review.

®Maharishi Ayur-Veda, Maharishi Transcendental Meditation, Transcendental Meditation, TM, TM-Sidhi, Maharishi Vedic Approach to Health, Maharishi Vedic Medicine, Maharishi Rejuvenation, Maharishi Gandharva Veda, Gandharva Veda Music, Maharishi Vedic Astrology, Maharishi Sthapatya Veda, Maharishi Jyotish, Maharishi Yagya, Maharishi Yoga, Maharishi Rasayana Program, Maharishi Vedic Vibration Technology, Instant Relief, Maharishi University of Management, Maharishi International University, Maharishi Vedic University, Maharishi Ayur-Veda University, Maharishi Vedic School, Maharishi Ayur-Veda School, Maharishi College of Vedic Medicine, Maharishi Ayur-Veda Health Center, Maharishi Medical Center, Maharishi Vedic Center, Maharishi Vedic Medical Center, Maharishi Vedic Sound, Maharishi Global Construction, Maharishi Vedic Science, and Maharishi Amrit Kalash are registered or common law trademarks licensed to Maharishi Vedic Education Development Corporation and used with permission.

ISBN 1-930051-55-7

We gratefully acknowledge permission to use material from the following published sources. The charts and text on pages 128, 153, 154, 157, and 160 are adapted from *Scientific Research on the Maharishi Transcendental Meditation and TM-Sidhi Programs: A Brief Summary of 500 Studies* (Fairfield, IA: Maharishi University of Management Press), ©1996 by Maharishi University of Management, and from *Scientific Research on the Maharishi Technology of the Unified Field: The Transcendental Meditation and TM-Sidhi Program* (Fairfield, IA: Maharishi International University Press), ©1988 by Maharishi International University. The charts and text on pages 129, 159, 197, 234, and 237 are adapted from *Summary of Research Findings* (Colorado Springs, CO: Maharishi Ayur-Veda Products International, Inc.), 1996.

Printed in the United States of America.

To His Holiness Maharishi Mahesh Yogi,
who has given us the knowledge of perfect health.

Contents

Acknowledgments

All that I have and all that I am is due to the infinite grace and love of my master, Maharishi Mahesh Yogi; my parents, Kameswaramma and Harischandra Reddy; my husband, Janardhan, and our children, Sundeep, Suma, and Hima; my paternal grandparents, Punnamma and Raghava Reddy Kondapalli; my maternal grandparents, Bhramaramba and Krishna Reddy Vatrapu; and my other immediate and world family members.

I would like to thank Professor Tony Nader, M.D., Ph.D, and Keith Wallace, Ph.D., for their guidance and wisdom throughout the writing of the book. Vaidya Hemant Gupta helped immensely with his careful research into the Vedic texts. I would especially like to thank senior editor Cynthia Lane for turning the manuscript into a book, Dick Kaynor and Mary Zeilbeck for editing, and Carol Kaynor and Martha Bright for copyediting. Thanks to Shepley Hansen for the cover design, Craig Ridgley for the layout and typesetting, and Jo Ann Gesner and Kathryn Peckman for the graphics. Thanks to Eva Herriott, Barnard Sherman, Geoffrey Hamilton, and all the others who helped in ways large and small.

A Note from the Author

The information included in this book is not in any way intended as a substitute for standard medical treatment. It is important that every patient follow the advice of his or her doctor for the treatment of any illness. Maharishi Vedic Medicine offers valuable complementary recommendations to supplement the advice of the primary care physician.

This book assumes that the reader has at least some acquaintance with Maharishi Vedic Medicine. Readers who are encountering this approach for the first time might enjoy referring to the more general introduction available in Dr. Reddy's first book (with Stan Kendz), *Forever Healthy—Introduction to Maharishi Ayur-Veda Health Care,* available from Samhita Productions.

I would like to pay tribute to the groundbreaking research into chronic disease being conducted by the Center for Natural Medicine and Prevention at Maharishi University of Management's College of Maharishi Vedic Medicine. Established in 1999 with a grant of $7.6 million from the National Institutes of Health (NIH) National Center for Complementary and Alternative Medicine, this research center is one of eleven recently established for the study of natural medicine throughout the U.S. It is the only one specializing in minority health, and focuses its research on the effectiveness of Maharishi Vedic Medicine in preventing and treating cardiovascular disease and other chronic disorders in high-risk and aging populations. In the future, the Center's scope will expand to include research on the cost effectiveness of Maharishi Vedic Medicine and pilot studies of modalities such as the effects of Maharishi Vedic Vibration Technology on ischemic heart disease.

The grant follows more than a decade of research on prevention-oriented natural medicine by Robert Schneider, M.D., Director of the Center, and his national team of collaborators. Earlier research grants of more than $10 million have been awarded Dr. Schneider and his team, who have published studies in American Heart Association journals *Hypertension* and *Stroke* showing that high blood pressure and atherosclerosis can be lowered or regressed with the Transcendental Meditation program, a well-known stress-reduction technique of Maharishi Vedic Medicine.

Additional research studies, published in periodicals such as the *American Journal of Cardiology, Psychosomatic Medicine, Ethnicity and Disease,* and *The American Journal of Managed Care,* have found that the modalities of Maharishi Vedic Medicine can reduce heart disease, decrease stress hormones, lower the need for health care utilization by 50 per cent, and promote longevity.

The Center includes collaborations with four major medical institutions and will serve as a training center for future researchers and physicians in the field of natural medicine. With this NIH-based support for research into modalities that enliven the body's inner intelligence, both the limitations of modern medicine and the promise of Maharishi Vedic Medicine is being further recognized by the medical community.

Foreword

by Jay Glaser, M.D.
Medical Director, Maharishi Ayur-Veda Medical Center
Lancaster, Massachusetts

In this well-organized and thoughtful book, Dr. Kumuda Reddy presents the one current, viable option for those suffering from chronic disease: Maharishi Vedic Medicine. The text is also a practical guide for health professionals who want to incorporate these principles into conventional medical practices. Dr. Reddy's presentation places this approach in its own category, distinct from many "alternative" or "complementary" therapies. Maharishi Vedic Medicine is a complete science with a theoretical framework and many practical applications. Dr. Reddy introduces us to its fascinating perspectives on human physiology and anatomy. Whether you are a health professional or simply someone interested in improving your health, you will find a broad yet specific range of practical interventions for chronic conditions.

In twelve years of our offering Maharishi Vedic Medicine as a primary treatment strategy, more than 6,000 patients have patronized the Maharishi Ayur-Veda Medical Center in Lancaster, Massachusetts. These patients are, by and large, not seeking a Maharishi Vedic Medicine specialist for conditions that they know are self-limiting, such as colds and poison ivy, or for problems that may require surgical intervention, such as appendicitis. Those are all "acute disorders." I am a firm believer in the utility of Western, allopathic approaches for acute conditions, but our patients come to us because our specialty is dealing with long-term problems that have defied Western medicine's "magic bullets"—problems of chronic disease. And, equally important, our patients are interested in learning to help themselves.

Chronic conditions are the end result of a process that usually has been going on for many years. The buildup of plaque in the coronary arteries, the erosion of the teeth due to plaque and gum disease, and the accumulating debris in the cytoplasm of an aging cell are all examples of such conditions that take a long time to develop and a long time to go away.

Unfortunately, modern medicine has failed to make significant progress against chronic disorders. Its palliative approaches, such as corticosteroids for inflammation, have often proven harmful. Back in the 1970s, in my early days as an attending physician in two Canadian hospitals, I quickly tired of treating patients on a superficial level. They viewed themselves as victims, and so did my profession. I couldn't make a difference in the underlying environmental factors behind their illnesses—stress, social and family disorder, poor diet, poor hygiene, etc.—that had a direct bearing on 95 per cent of the disorders I was seeing. It was a great pleasure and relief, as a physician, to discover that this gaping lack in modern medicine could be filled by Maharishi Vedic Medicine, whose treatments have proven successful not only in *treating* chronic disease, but in *preventing* it—while remaining free of harmful side effects. This is a remarkable achievement by today's standards.

In our own clinic we have seen dramatic improvements in a wide range of disorders, including neurological ones such as headache and insomnia. One common, visible result of our therapies is that our patients *look and feel younger, healthier, more vital.* This is because Maharishi Vedic Medicine's focus is not so much to treat particular symptoms as to correct distortions in the expression of the intelligence within each cell. Put more simply, the idea is to get at the real root of the problem. By "rewriting the body's software," as it were, we see spontaneous reductions in symptomatic complaints even among those who have been suffering the longest.

Chronic disease is the end result of an insidious process occurring over many years, often invisibly. Chronic disease is unlike traumatic injuries or acute disorders, which arise suddenly and respond to the body's natural mechanisms of self-repair. A young man suffering from a motorcycle crash with severe abrasions, fractures, contusions, blood loss, unstable vital signs and pain may be told by the doctors with genuine confidence, "Don't worry, you're going to be fine," because they know that his recuperative capacities are greater than the injuries. But their prognosis for the woman in the next room who feels "just fine" following an episode of chest pain may not be as rosy, because they know that underlying the problem is a persistent, ongoing imbalance that they are not well-equipped to eliminate.

The most chronic of all chronic diseases is aging, which is the expression of accumulated stress. My experience both as a medical doctor and as a specialist in Maharishi Vedic Medicine is that this and other chronic diseases can only be treated successfully by enlivening the underlying intelligence responsible for our biological existence. Maharishi Vedic Medicine works its magic on the level of this process.

As you explore this text, you will see that we are intimately connected to the entire universe, which is maintained in perfect balance by Nature's incredible organizing power. Dr. Reddy has given us a handbook to return to the perfection that is naturally within every one of us.

Author Foreword

For many years, I was a faculty member and anesthesiologist at Albany Medical College, practicing the conventional medical approach to health care. For the past twelve years or more, however, I have devoted myself to spreading the knowledge and benefits of Maharishi Vedic Medicine. What prompted me to make this change? I did this because I came to realize the importance of a holistic approach to maintaining health that took into account our relationship to the natural world around us. We are one with nature. Because of our intimate connection with nature and the entire cosmos, we need natural and holistic medicine. It is the need of our time, and in my experience, no other medicine has proven to be as natural, comprehensive, and holistic as Maharishi Vedic Medicine.

"Avert the danger which has not yet come." This is the basic principle of prevention from the classic Vedic texts. And the earlier we start, the better. Everyone should know that it is not necessary to suffer anymore. You have a choice in your life. By making the right choices in your lifestyle and diet, it is possible to remove the mistakes that lead to discomfort and disease. It is a simple but very effective approach to good health for you and your whole family.

Using Maharishi Vedic Medicine, I have been fortunate to have helped thousands of patients live healthier, happier, and longer lives. I hope when you read this book that you too will take the first steps on the road to perfect health.

With my very best wishes,

Kumuda Reddy, M.D.

CONQUERING
CHRONIC DISEASE
THROUGH MAHARISHI VEDIC MEDICINE

PART I
Establishing a Reference Point for Health

Establishing a Reference Point for Health

Chronic disease is the great medical problem of our time. Nearly half the population suffers from chronic disease, and in many ways our modern medical system has failed them. Modern medicine has in fact become fragmented. It has increasingly put its focus on the treatment of disease and its many symptoms, rather than on creating healthy people. In so doing, it may have lost track of what health really is.

When researchers study the nature of disease rather than health, they see many individual factors and isolated symptoms. They see the intricacies of disease in such detail that some illnesses may appear too complicated to cure. However, they are learning about sickness, not health, so the possibility of relatively simple and permanent cures too often eludes them.

This book provides a new paradigm, a new reference point for health. Maharishi Vedic Medicine treats chronic disease by successfully removing its deepest cause. In that process, it awakens the innate, inner healing intelligence of the body and brings health to every part of life, transforming chronic disease into the joy of living the full potential of mind and body.

Chapter 1 discusses the dramatic problem of chronic disease and explains how the Maharishi Vedic Approach to Health℠ offers effective solutions. Chapter 2 takes a visionary look at the state of human health before disease begins. It explores the underlying intelligence that pilots the mind-body and gives rise to its various complex systems and organs. You'll see how mind, body, emotions, and environment are all part of the wholeness we call health.

In Chapter 3, you'll look at the structure of the healthy human body from the perspective of Maharishi Vedic Medicine. With the concept of genuine health as the reference point, we can begin the discussion of disease.

CHAPTER 1

Chronic Disease Is Mankind's Greatest Enemy

"Maharishi Vedic Approach to Health is destined to create a disease-free, healthy, enlightened society."
—*Maharishi Mahesh Yogi*[1]

It was only a small part of an article in a professional journal for doctors, yet it alarmed Americans from all walks of life. The article, published in the November 1993 issue of the *Journal of the American Medical Association*[2] (JAMA) stated that 100 million people in this country suffer from chronic disease. For a nation that sees itself as a world leader in health care, it spends more than one trillion dollars on health care annually, and serves as a model for many developing countries. This statistic was a bombshell. In effect, we learned that nearly one of every two Americans is chronically ill.

The story contained more shocking news. Thirty-nine million Americans suffer from more than one chronic condition. As physicians often observe, one disease leads to another. Rather than improving with modern medical treatment, this situation is actually worsening. The percentage of Americans suffering from chronic disease has doubled in this century.

In 1935, when the first National Health Survey was conducted, less than 22 per cent of the population had a chronic disease. In 1987, when the survey for this article was conducted, 45 per cent of noninstitutionalized Americans suffered from one or more chronic diseases. Based on the 1997 rates of chronic disease and population growth rates, the number of persons of all ages with chronic conditions will increase to 148 million by 2030.

What It Means to Have a Chronic Disease

What is chronic disease? The dictionary defines it as a major disorder that lasts for a long period of time or continually reappears. In our culture, "chronic" usually means incurable. Chronic conditions range from life-threatening illnesses, such as coronary heart disease and cancer, to life-diminishing disorders, such as chronic fatigue, arthritis, and migraine headaches.

Nearly every family in America is now affected. Chronic disease not only causes tremendous suffering to the person involved, requiring huge expenditures of money, energy, and time just to manage it, but also strains family relationships and drains earning power and job productivity. When chronic illness strikes even one person, it can have a devastating impact on other family members. People live longer now, yet family sizes—or the potential pool of caregivers—are smaller. The chances of finding yourself in the role of caregiver are greater than ever before.

Today's Health Care Does Not Address Chronic Disease . . .

At one time, infectious disease was the greatest threat to health. Plagues and scourges swept across the globe, killing huge numbers of people in a matter of weeks. The national health care system had to be prepared to respond to large-scale disasters and medical crises. In the Western world, this situation started to change as early as the 1920s, when health statisticians began noticing that chronic (long-term) illnesses were replacing infectious diseases as the dominant health care challenge.

"Our health care system remains firmly rooted in episodic and acute care, but it is unlikely to continue this way in the next century,"[3] pointed out the authors of the JAMA article. They observed that there is a huge gap between the prevalence of chronic diseases today and the antiquated nature of our health care system, which is not designed to deal with them.

Lack of access to medical care presents another disturbing aspect of the spread of chronic disease. Thirty-five per cent of U.S. citizens are now either insufficiently covered or have no medical insurance at all. In 1987, direct health care costs for people who had chronic disorders accounted for three-fourths of the U.S. government's health care expenditures, amounting to $659 billion. If current trends continue, projected direct costs will rise to $798 billion.

. . . And May Be Hazardous to Your Health

If nearly half the people in the most advanced medical system of the world are chronically ill, then at the very least, it's a sign that this system is not as successful at promoting health as it should be. However, the problem is worse than that. The medical system may actually be contributing to disease. Everyone is aware of the miracles performed by modern drugs and technologies. What is less well known is that in many cases these powerful therapies are actually the cause of future chronic conditions.

Iatrogenic disease is the name for disorders that are created as the result of the harmful side effects of modern drugs, diagnostic procedures and surgery. Such a great number of patients suffer injury from medical treatment in the United States that iatrogenic disease accounts for more deaths than all other accidents combined. According to the *Journal of the American Medical Association*, 180,000 people die in the United States alone each year as a result of iatrogenic injury, which is the equivalent of three jumbo jet crashes every two days.[4]

The growing need for stronger and stronger antibiotics represents another significant health problem. Antibiotics have been used to eliminate microorganisms, but in the process, more resistant strains of bacteria have developed. Researchers around the world are concerned that we may have epidemics that cannot be restrained by drugs. In fact, this may have already started happening. New strains of tuberculosis are emerging that are resistant to the current drugs.[5] Even worse, as the microorganisms get stronger and more resistant, the drugs to kill them must be increasingly potent, posing a risk to the individuals receiving the drugs.

Antibiotics are frequently overused. For instance, they are regularly prescribed to treat problems such as urinary tract infections, even though antibiotics are completely useless if the problem is not caused by bacteria. Taking the drugs only weakens the body's immunity, making it more susceptible to disease in the future. Unfortunately, antibiotics are wrongly prescribed for many diseases, as a rather startling statistic reveals. "Doctors write as many as 12 million unnecessary antibiotic prescriptions yearly for colds, upper-respiratory-tract infections, and bronchitis. The drugs do little or nothing to fight the viral illnesses."[6]

Help for Chronic Disease Is Available

When I see patients in my practice, I have come to feel that humankind has no greater enemy than chronic disease. Nothing else is as disruptive to normal life and causes so much suffering, not only for the person who has the heart attack or stroke, but also for the family and other caretakers. At the same time, I have found no greater conqueror of chronic disease than Maharishi Vedic Medicine.

Patients come to me with a wide range of chronic disorders, such as arthritis, chronic fatigue, sinusitis, persistent allergies, irritable bowel syndrome, hypertension, lower back pain, weight gain or loss, anxiety or depression, sleep disorder, substance abuse, migraine headaches, and menstrual or menopausal problems. I have found that these diseases respond remarkably well to the natural treatments of Maharishi Vedic Medicine. What is most important is that these treatments get to the root cause of disease and eradicate it at its source, provided the disease is not too advanced.

At age 52, Mary's* blood pressure was at such a dangerous level, 240 over 140, that her doctors told her not to exert herself in any way. It was just a matter of time, they said, before a heart attack or stroke would strike her down. The worst thing was that no one could help her. At her urging, her doctor sent her to a special hospital in her area, where extensive diagnostic tests were conducted for four days. The diagnosis—they found no organic cause for Mary's high blood pressure. The recommendation— Mary should take antidepressants to cope with her incurable condition.

At that time, Mary was taking blood pressure medicine, which had no effect in lowering her blood pressure. Worse, it was creating extreme fatigue, aches in her body, dizziness, headaches and dry mouth. When she asked her doctor to decrease the dosage, he told her that he could no longer help her and not to come back.

By the time Mary came to me, she was frightened and angry. "I felt like there was no hope for me," she says. "I couldn't believe that people were turning me away. I knew that I wasn't ready to die."

When I explained the natural therapies of Maharishi Vedic Medicine, she actually started to cry with relief. That was four years ago, and her blood pressure today is only 140/90. Even though that is still a moderately high level for most people, for Mary it is a dramatic improvement. Today Mary can do everything and anything she wants, including mountain hiking and enjoying a new relationship.

"The most wonderful thing is that now I don't think about dying," she says. "Instead I think about growing old."

Diagnosed with fibromyositis, John, age 36, was suffering from

-----

*Patient names used through this book have been changed to protect their privacy.

9

such severe pain, tightness, and stiffness in his neck and back muscles that he had decided to shut down his chiropractic practice for a few months to recover. Associated symptoms of chronic fatigue and tension headaches, plus a thirty-year history of bronchial asthma, had already forced him to cut back his patient load over the previous six months.

After receiving treatments from Maharishi Vedic Medicine, John improved dramatically. Within six weeks, his backache had completely disappeared and the joint and shoulder pains were much milder. He experienced only one headache in the first six weeks and reported much less fatigue. His asthma improved so much that he used his inhaler only once a day. The improvement was so profound that he was able to resume his full-time practice and continues to make progress each week.

Another patient, Laurie, age 40, had always felt basically healthy. Then she hit her late 30s and started having repetitive ovarian cysts. Birth control pills didn't seem to help with the severe pain and a feeling of hormonal imbalance. When her gynecologist suggested surgery to remove her ovary, she decided to seek alternative treatments. She read about Maharishi Vedic Medicine in a book and was drawn to its broad approach to women's health and hormonal cycles. She was pleasantly surprised to find a physician trained in Maharishi Vedic Medicine near her home. After discussing it with her gynecologist, who was open to the idea, she decided to come to our clinic.

When she started the Maharishi Vedic Medicine treatments, not only did her cysts disappear, but her overall health improved dramatically. "I'm not having the cysts, but even better, my body feels much more in balance emotionally and physically," she said. "I feel better than I did at age eighteen. I'm a high-energy person, sometimes too high-energy, and it would sometimes get in the way. Now there are days when I feel like I could go forever, and I'm not driving myself crazy by running around and feeling frantic."

"I liked the whole approach," Laurie stated. "You don't just go in there and say, 'Hey, I have a pain in my right ovary, so let's fix it.' Instead, she [Dr. Reddy] asked me what was going on with my life and my family, what was my lifestyle like. She looked at me as a whole person rather than a disease."

I have successfully treated many hundreds of patients like these in my private practice, as have many other physicians trained in Maharishi Vedic Medicine throughout the world. You may be wondering how the natural therapies of Maharishi Vedic Medicine can cure such long-term, serious problems when Western medicine has had little or no effect. Maharishi Vedic Medicine is so effective because it views health and disease in a completely different way from modern medicine.

The Uniqueness of Maharishi Vedic Medicine

When people become seriously ill, they often find themselves asking, "Why me?" Many times patients come to me in a state of shock, confusion, and anger, wondering how this could have happened to them.

One of the first things that helps a person start on the road to recovery is the realization that ill health does not just happen. Causes exist and they yield effects. Some of the causes are not easily controlled. They may lie in genes, for example, or in environmental pollutants. However, you yourself can influence many of the other causes. Much chronic disease begins with the choices a person makes every day—the choice to eat healthy or unhealthy foods, to avoid or to court stress, to listen to the body when it cries for rest or to force it to function even when fatigued. We call these wrong choices "violations of Natural Law," and such violations, over the long run, create disease.

This may strike you as a harsh way of speaking to someone who is sick. However, when people recognize that earlier choices may have contributed to or even caused illness, they can also see that making different choices will help them to become healthy again. Knowledge increases your choices and brings you to greater freedom.

Maharishi Vedic Medicine is based on complete knowledge of how to live in harmony with the Laws of Nature. The word *Veda* means "knowledge," total knowledge of Natural Law. Maharishi Vedic Medicine was brought to light in recent years by Maharishi Mahesh Yogi, who is best known as the founder of the Transcendental Meditation® (TM®) technique.

When someone is sick, each day may feel dark. The simplest way to dispel darkness is to turn on the light, in this case the light provided by knowledge. The Maharishi Vedic Approach to Health is based on a profound and comprehensive knowledge that is not yet commonly accepted or understood by allopathic medicine.

Focusing on Prevention

Knowledge of how to live in harmony with Natural Law gives you the tools to prevent disease from happening in the first place. It's an ironic fact that in America, more than 60 per cent of the money spent on health care is spent during the last six months of a person's life, when the body is essentially beyond repair.

When disease develops, its cause has already been present for quite a while. Drop by drop, pathogenic influences create imbalance over a long period. Like a window accumulating dirt, the dust and grime build up bit by bit. It's not just one piece of dirt that makes a window cloudy. All the dust and dirt together gradually make it unable to allow in light.

Doctors everywhere know that at least 50 per cent of disease is preventable. Unhealthy habits such as poor diet, inadequate exercise, smoking and alcohol abuse contribute to disease, as does the stress of contemporary life. Yet our modern health care system does not tell people how to break these habits, how to change their lifestyles to create health instead of disease. Maharishi Vedic Medicine identifies not only these most obvious causal factors but also many other behaviors and routines that create imbalance in the mind-body. But even more important, it provides technologies for bringing people into harmony with Natural Law, so that their behavior becomes totally life-supporting. They learn how to avoid the mistakes that cause ill health. In this way, Maharishi Vedic Medicine effectively helps people to prevent disease long before it has blossomed into full-blown symptoms.

Holistic and Individualized Treatment Approaches

Maharishi Vedic Medicine is both profound and comprehensive in its effects, in part because it is based on a holistic model of health and offers a wide range of treatment modalities. It takes into account forty aspects of inner intelligence, most of which are not considered in modern medicine. Maharishi Vedic Medicine is successful because it enlivens all forty of these areas of inner intelligence, restoring balance to mind, body, emotions and the environment. Moreover, all of its approaches enliven Nature's intelligence, or consciousness, which is at the basis of all aspects of both the structure and function of our minds, emotions, and bodies. This makes each approach holistic in and of itself.

Maharishi Vedic Medicine treats the whole person, and each angle of treatment is individualized. A basic tenet of Maharishi Vedic Medicine is that each person must be diagnosed to determine the specific imbalances producing his problem. In addition, it assesses each individual's constitution and tendencies. Two people with the same symptoms will not necessarily have the same treatment. The symptoms for a disease such as bronchial asthma could be caused by entirely different imbalances in different people. Therapy is highly personalized. The physician takes into account each person's mental, physical and emotional tendencies as well as his environment. The treatment program is prescribed for the individual, not the disease.

An entire section of this book is devoted to describing the

therapeutic modalities, but we'll briefly describe the major approaches here.

Enlivening Consciousness

When Laura came to me with her ovarian cysts, I suggested she take a course in the Transcendental Meditation technique, because it is the most powerful method for enlivening consciousness—the source of the mind-body's intelligence—and bringing the entire system back into balance. Once she started to meditate, her body's own healing responses were spontaneously enlivened, making all treatment modalities more effective. The Transcendental Meditation technique is really the cornerstone of Maharishi Vedic Medicine, and it has been shown in hundreds of scientific research studies to reduce stress and create better mental, emotional, and physical health, enhancing all areas of life.

Purifying and Balancing the Body

For some conditions, a physician trained in Maharishi Vedic Medicine might prescribe a combination of herbal formulas, herbalized massage therapies, and internal cleansing programs—all part of Maharishi Rejuvenation therapy—to detoxify the body and remove the blocks to the flow of Nature's intelligence in the body. Laura needed some specific remedies for her physical system, to stop the pain and the growth of the cysts. For this, she was given a special diet to recreate physiological balance. Herbal compounds also helped balance the mind-body system and reestablish the diseased area's connection with Nature's (and the body's) underlying intelligence. Many other approaches to purify and balance the body can be used, including Yoga postures.

Adjusting the Behavior

Behavior is also part of Maharishi Vedic Medicine. The times when we wake up, go to bed, and eat can all affect our well-being and energy levels. The Vedic daily routine and seasonal routines help bring individual biorhythms into harmony with Nature's rhythms, rather than fighting against or trying to ignore them.

Balancing the Near Environment

Environmental effects represent a fascinating area of health that is largely ignored today. In truth, the environment constantly affects our physical and mental well-being, which is why Maharishi Vedic Medicine is concerned about the design of the buildings in which we live and work. We have all heard of "sick building syndrome," where the materials and design of modern buildings have actually caused allergies, asthma, and severe headaches. One of the approaches of Maharishi Vedic Medicine, called Sthapatya Veda, goes deeply into the health effects of the orientation, design, proportion and positioning of buildings. It explains how to build structures that are in harmony with the Laws of Nature and the land—structures that can actually improve health and happiness in those who occupy them.

Balancing the Distant Environment

The environment beyond our homes also affects our health—not only the environmental toxins and pressures of modern life that bring so much stress to our bodies and minds, but also the cycles of Nature. These include rhythmic motions of the moon, sun, and planets. The effects of these cycles are described in the approach of Maharishi Vedic Medicine called the Maharishi Jyotish program, which also provides recommendations and procedures to mitigate negative influences that can cause ill health or strengthen positive influences that support good health.

Balancing Collective Health

Finally, the influence of collective health, or the health of society, is a key part of Maharishi Vedic Medicine. Crime, famine, war, and disruptions in the economy are all expressions of ill health in the collective body we call society. Each of these problems in society affects individual health. Maharishi Vedic Medicine includes techniques to create balance in collective as well as individual health. The goal is to create a world where no person will be threatened by negative influences from others, and every person will contribute to a healthy and harmonious atmosphere for everyone.

Treating the Deepest Source of the Problem

While Western medicine tends to focus on identifying and eliminating isolated symptoms one by one, Maharishi Vedic Medicine seeks to identify the primary cause of the many symptoms. By eliminating deep, underlying imbalances rather than just superficial symptoms, Maharishi Vedic Medicine provides much more effective methods to create long-lasting and real relief from chronic problems.

Certainly in Western medicine we have analyzed the causes of disease, as well as the manifestations and complications. However, we have never before understood the fundamental principle that disease originates and therefore must be treated at a profound, subtle level of the mind-body system. A recent conversation with one of my medical colleagues, who also has been trained in Maharishi Vedic Medicine, comes to mind. After reading a recent research article on irritable bowel syndrome, she commented, "So many hundreds of research studies have been conducted on just this one problem. Western physicians know all the causes of irritable bowel syndrome, know all of the symptoms that can manifest, and have many treatment approaches. Yet none of these treatments have a very happy outcome." Sadly enough, physicians would be the first to admit that the symptom-based tools available to them are rarely effective in treating this particular chronic ailment.

It is important to state that this book is not meant as a replacement for Western medical treatment. As a former anesthesiologist, I would be the first to recognize the great advances in drugs and technologies, which are remarkable in their ability to save lives in many situations. Maharishi Vedic Medicine embraces everything that is useful and helpful in medicine. We do not denounce conventional medicine, but instead we use it as needed. This natural, comprehensive health care is a perfect complement to any necessary conventional medical interventions. At no time in this book are we advocating that a person with a serious chronic disease stop his medication or treatment without the advice of his medical doctor.

Some of the Chronic Diseases
Successfully Treated by Maharishi Vedic Medicine

Allergies	Benign prostatic hyperplasia
Constipation	Chronic liver disease
Digestive disorders	Gallstones
Coronary heart disease	Hyperacidity
Hypertension	Peptic ulcer
Chronic bronchitis	Irritable bowel syndrome
Bronchial asthma	Inflammatory bowel disease
Chronic sinusitis	Menstrual problems
Chronic headache	Menopausal syndrome
Rheumatoid arthritis	Depression
Osteoarthritis	Chronic anxiety
Chronic fatigue	Insomnia
Chronic back pain	Connective tissue diseases
Diabetes (non-insulin dependent)	Thyroid disease (hypo- and hyperthyroidism)
Weight problems	Alzheimer's disease
Psoriasis	Parkinson's disease
Eczema	Multiple sclerosis
Chronic kidney disease	

In critical conditions, when quick intervention is needed to save a life, conventional medicine has been very effective. When someone is sick we give them whatever medicine works to stabilize their condition.

On the other hand, I have experienced first-hand that Maharishi Vedic Medicine can serve as a marvelous adjunct to conventional medical care. Most of my patients have come to me because in some way Western medicine has failed them. They have tried the modern approaches, but for their particular chronic conditions, the available drugs and therapies just haven't worked. They have often expressed confusion, betrayal and anger because their doctors have not been able to cure them.

One of my greatest joys in life has been to offer these patients both immediate and long-term relief with the natural, holistic therapies of Maharishi Vedic Medicine. These treatments—which include stress reduction techniques, lifestyle changes, dietary changes, exercise, herbal compounds targeted for specific disorders, and other natural therapies—produce an overall balance that allows patients to begin functioning as healthier people and break the gripping pattern of ill health that has plagued them for so long. In the following chapters, you will meet many more people who are conquering chronic disease through Maharishi Vedic Medicine.

CHAPTER 2

Health and the Body's Inner Intelligence

"A perfectly healthy person lives in the state of enlightenment, with the spontaneous ability to use the total organizing power of Natural Law to accomplish any goal in a natural way without strain. Ill health is fundamentally due to violation of Natural Law caused by lack of knowledge of Natural Law. Lack of knowledge of Natural Law weakens the individual and creates stress in society."
    —*Maharishi Mahesh Yogi*[7]

You cannot understand disease unless you first understand health. One way health can be defined is freedom from chronic disease, a perspective that seems to be based on survival. Maharishi Vedic Medicine offers a more expanded definition, because it aims for an ideal state of health. Here, perfect health is not just the absence of disease, it is a state of functioning that the Vedic seers called "enlightenment." This definition takes into account the whole person—consciousness, mind, emotions, behavior, and environment—in addition to the body. In fact, the Sanskrit word for health is *swasthya*, meaning wholeness.

The Vedic texts describe enlightenment as a state of perfect balance in mind and body. The person who enjoys this state lives in perfect harmony with Nature and with everyone around him. Such a person thinks clearly, creatively, and expansively. He or she experiences success and fulfillment in every area of life. Enlightened individuals act in a way that is simultaneously helpful to themselves, their families, societies, nations, and the world. In other words, these people enjoy perfect health and balance not only in their bodies, but also in every arena of life. They live in harmony with the entire creation. To experience perfect health, then, is to enjoy the balance, orderliness and power inherent in Nature itself.

The Underlying Field of Nature's Intelligence

Maharishi Vedic Medicine considers the body as an integrated expression of Nature's intelligence, rather than as a machine with many loosely related parts to repair. The Vedic texts describe a unified field of pure intelligence underlying all of Nature's manifest expressions. This concept may seem strange or new, but it is highly similar to current theories used by unified field physicists. In the Vedic paradigm, the same intelligence that keeps the planets moving in their orbits and manages the interconnecting web of life in a forest or on an ocean floor also orchestrates the functioning of billions of cells, millions of functions, and hundreds of systems in the human body. This means that each human mind also arises from this unified field of pure, creative intelligence.

Think of the dynamism and power of a river, which can generate enough electricity to light whole cities. What if that power and dynamism were unlimited, infinite? The unified field underlying all of creation is a field of unlimited intelligence, energy, creativity and organizing power. It exists at the basis of every human life and everyone can access it. If you get in touch with this infinite resource of power and bliss that is the fundamental source of all thought and action, then you can restore perfect health to every layer of the mind-body.

The human body is an expression of the same creative intelligence that runs the universe. This basic understanding—that an underlying intelligence governs the body's functioning—is the main difference between Maharishi Vedic Medicine and Western approaches.

The Body Is Consciousness

Most people usually think of their physical bodies when they define the word health. Yet no one would doubt that the bones, skin, blood, hair, nails, and muscles that make up the body are only part of his or her nature. The subtle and more powerful aspects—mind, feelings, and consciousness itself—are also part of a person. The physical body is only one portion of the whole person, one small part of the total sum. Maharishi Vedic Medicine defines our true nature as a combination of consciousness, mind, and body.

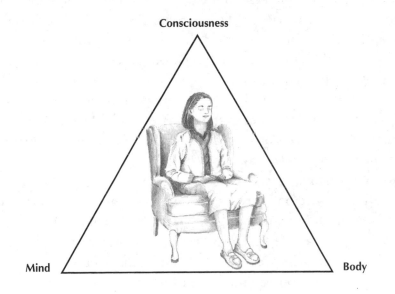

What is consciousness? You've already read about the underlying field of pure intelligence that gives rise to all of creation. You can experience this field of limitless intelligence as pure awareness or being, the mind's fundamental inner wakefulness without an object of experience. This experience, available during the Transcendental Meditation practice, lets you discover the unmanifest field of unlimited potential and perfect orderliness that is your own essential nature, and which permeates the entire universe—including the human body.

Imagine being in a movie theater before the movie starts. A large, blank white screen sits in front of you and you may or may not think about it. (Probably not.) Once the movie begins, the images totally cover the screen. It is lost to view and to immediate experience. The movie totally obscures the screen, yet if it wasn't there, you could not see the movie. The only way to see the screen again is to remove the film.

Consciousness is like the blank white screen. Without that pure awareness, that essential liveliness or wakefulness of the mind, you could have no experience. The content of daily life—from vague thoughts and feelings to concrete objects and complex events— "covers" or hides the underlying field of consciousness, just as the movie hides the screen. You forget it is there, even though without it, you could have no experience. When you transcend normal, everyday mental activity during the Transcendental Meditation technique, all the objects of perception—all the pieces of information the senses take in—are transcended and you can unite with your most fundamental nature—pure consciousness.

Your mind and body are an expression of this field of pure potential. You could say that when consciousness manifests into matter, it appears as the human system (as well as many other systems). Consciousness creates and maintains every facet of the mind and body. Consequently, when something is wrong with the body, it means something is wrong with its connection to its fundamental constituent, consciousness. With this model of the human body, it is easy to see that sustaining an unobstructed experience of pure consciousness, the body's deepest organizing principle, is the most basic requirement for health.

In today's culture, people often identify with their bodies. The underlying field of Nature's intelligence, which operates the entire body from the level of the DNA, is most often unrecognized and neglected. Just as the sap of a tree nourishes all the colorful leaves, branches, and trunk of the tree, so the intelligence of the body nourishes and orders the work of every cell, yet both remain unseen and generally overlooked.

The Power of the Mind

During the past thirty years, extensive research has shown that the mind is intimately connected with the body and that many diseases originate in the mind. These are called psychosomatic diseases. In Maharishi Vedic Medicine, the mind-body connection has been recognized for thousands of years. In fact, symptoms are always described in terms of their mental and physical characteristics. All disease is perceived as caused by the mind and body together.

In the Vedic view of health, mind is an abstract value that expresses itself through the senses and brain, which allow you to experience the world through hearing, tasting, touching, smelling, and seeing. In this model, the body is the metabolic end-product of mind. You metabolize your thoughts through your body. A stressed thought creates a stressed molecule. You need to create contentment and the warmth of bliss. Maharishi Vedic Medicine bridges the gulf between consciousness and the body and smooths their connection.

In Maharishi Vedic Medicine, a contented, happy mind is an indication and precursor of health. In fact, a person cannot be considered healthy unless the mind is full of bliss. Fear, anger, jealousy, and other negative emotions are signs and precursors of imbalance or ill health.

Natural Law and the Physiology

This chapter explored the field of Nature's intelligence, which is also called *Veda*. Veda is the totality of Natural Law, the unified state of all the Laws of Nature. The Veda and Vedic Literature contain complete knowledge of all the impulses, or Laws of Nature, that create and maintain the universe.

The many different impulses of Nature's intelligence, called Natural Laws, give order and direction to every facet of the manifest creation and the human mind-body. Your inner intelligence operates and coordinates different systems and organs in the body. When this intelligence takes on different qualities in the context of creation, it gives rise to different parts of the body.

This has been brought to light in a recent discovery by Professor Tony Nader, M.D., Ph.D., in which he found direct correlations between the many facets of Vedic Literature and the myriad areas and systems of the human body. The same impulses of pure intelligence or consciousness that give rise to different aspects of the human body are expressed in the forty aspects of the Vedic Literature. Six of these forty texts deal explicitly with medicine and health, and are known collectively as *Ayur-Veda,* literally "knowledge of the lifespan." The best known of these six texts is the *Charaka Samhita,* to which you'll see many references in this book.

The six Ayurvedic texts were the first to receive Maharishi's attention in his revival of Vedic medicine. Initially presented as the Maharishi Ayur-Veda® health program*, this system has now incorporated all forty aspects of Veda and Vedic Literature, thanks to Dr. Nader's discovery. While the Ayurvedic texts form the core of Maharishi Vedic Medicine's diagnostic and treatment modalities, each one of all forty aspects of Vedic Literature expresses a different value of Natural Law. Each offers a unique contribution to understanding and pefecting all forty major aspects of the body's inner intelligence.

The practical significance of Dr. Nader's discovery cannot be underestimated. First, it illustrates that every person is a living,

---

*See Dr. Reddy's first book, *Forever Healthy—An Introduction to Maharishi Ayur-Veda Health Care.*

Forty Aspects of Veda in Human Physiology

Aspect of Vedic Literature	Quality of Natural Law	Expression in Physiology
Rik Veda	Holistic—Dynamic Silence	Whole Physiology
Sama Veda	Flowing Wakefulness, Flowing	Sensory Systems
Yajur-Veda	Offering and Creating	Processing Systems
Atharva Veda	Reverberating Wholeness, Reverberating	Motor Systems
Shiksha	Expressing	Autonomic Ganglia
Kalpa	Transforming	Limbic System
Vyakarana	Expanding	Hypothalamus
Nirukta	Self-referral	Autonomic Nervous System and Pituitary Gland
Chhandas	Measuring and Quantifying	Neurohormones, Neurotransmitters
Jyotisha	All-knowing	Basal Ganglia, Deep-seated Nuclei
Nyaya	Distinguishing and Deciding	Thalamus
Vaisheshika	Specifying	Cerebellum
Samkhya	Enumerating	Cells, Tissues, Organs—Types and Categories
Yoga	Unifying	Cerebral Cortex
Karma Mimansa	Analyzing	Central Nervous System
Vedanta	Lively Absolute (Living Wholeness—I-ness or Being)	Integrated Functioning of the Nervous System
Gandharva Veda	Integrating and Harmonizing	Cycles and Rhythms
Dhanur-Veda	Invincible and Progressive	Biochemistry, Enzymes, Immune System, Vertebral Column
Sthapatya Veda	Establishing	Anatomy
Harita Samhita	Nourishing	Venous and Biliary Systems
Bhela Samhita	Differentiating	Lymphatic System, Glial Cells
Kashyapa Samhita	Equivalency	Arterial System
Charaka Samhita	Balancing—Holding Together and Supporting	Cell Nucleus
Sushruta Samhita	Separating	Cytoplasm, Cell Organelles
Vagbhata Samhita	Communication and Eloquence	Cytoskeleton, Cell Membrane
Madhava Nidan Samhita	Diagnosing	Mesodermal Tissues
Sharngadhara Samhita	Synthesizing	Endodermal Tissues
Bhava-Prakasha Samhita	Enlightening	Ectodermal Tissues
Upanishad	Transcending	Ascending Tracts of Central Nervous System
Aranyaka	Stirring	Fasciculi Proprii
Brahmana	Structuring	Descending Tracts of Central Nervous System
Itihasa	Blossoming of Totality	Voluntary Motor and Sensory Projections
Purana	Ancient and Eternal	Great Intermediate Net
Smriti	Memory	Memory Systems, Reflexes
Rik Veda Pratishakhya	All-pervading Wholeness	Cerebral Cortex, Layer 1
Shukla-Yajur-Veda Pratishakhya	Silencing, Sharing, and Spreading	Cerebral Cortex, Layer 2
Atharva Veda Pratishakhya	Unfolding	Cerebral Cortex, Layer 5
Atharva Veda Pratishakhya (Chaturadhyayi)	Dissolving	Cerebral Cortex, Layer 6
Krishna-Yajur-Veda Pratishakhya	Omnipresent	Cerebral Cortex, Layer 3
Sama Veda Pratishakhya	Unmanifesting the Parts but Manifesting the Whole	Cerebral Cortex, Layer 4

breathing, talking embodiment of Veda—a storehouse of pure knowledge, pure intelligence, pure orderliness, happiness, and organizing power. Every person has a blueprint for living perfect health and a perfect life within his or her own body.

Second, it provides the basis for a comprehensive health care system that truly enlivens and nourishes every aspect of the human consciousness, mind, body and environment from the most profound level of life. Maharishi Vedic Medicine, by providing practical approaches to match the forty different aspects of the Veda and Vedic Literature expressed in the human body, is truly holistic, bringing every detail of human life into the realm of health and happiness.

You Are Not Your Disease

In this chapter, you have seen that Maharishi Vedic Medicine considers the whole person, not just the disease. After all, when something is wrong with your arm, you don't send just your arm to the doctor! Moreover, from this perspective, your body is not simply a solid, material mass of bone, muscle, and skin. Instead, your mind and body are expressions of Nature's intelligence, power, bliss, wholeness, dynamism, energy and balance.

It's important to grasp this not only from the viewpoint of health, but also of disease. If the human being that you call yourself is not just a body, but an expression of the infinite power of Nature, then you are not just your disease. So many people, when they are faced with a chronic disease, become identified with it. Many times patients start to think of themselves as a heart attack patient, a cancer patient, a diabetic. This is compounded by the fact that medical doctors are trained to focus on disease, and sometimes their patients become known only by their diseases. People tend to lose sight of the fact that their consciousness, or inner intelligence, rules the body not the other way around. They start to think of disease as normal. Disease becomes their reference point for judging health.

Any health care system based on partial knowledge will only yield partial health. If you want to have perfect health, you must base your health care on complete knowledge. The Veda contains the total knowledge of life as pure potential, just as a seed contains the total potential, in unmanifest form, of the whole tree. Everything that the tree can become is there in the seed. In Maharishi Vedic Medicine, every treatment helps establish a reference point for health in the stable, non-changing field of pure consciousness or pure knowledge, the field of the Veda. This field of *Being*, which contains within itself the total potential of Natural Law—the seed for the entire tree of creation—is the foundation for perfect health. A clear, unbroken experience of it is the criterion for perfect health. As you begin to unfold the infinite potential for healing within, happiness, intelligence, mental clarity and optimal physical health become your daily experience.

CHAPTER 3

The Structure of the Healthy Human Body

"Every aspect of the physiology is managed by these specific qualities of intelligence within it, and the Law that maintains precision and order in the performing intelligence of Nature provides a common ground for harmonizing all life."

—*Maharishi Mahesh Yogi*[8]

You now know the most important principle of Maharishi Vedic Medicine—your body is an expression of Nature's pure intelligence. It is constructed of the same intelligence that composes every atom in creation. As the *Charaka Samhita* puts it, "All the material and spiritual phenomena of the universe are present in the individual. Similarly all those present in the individual are also contained in the universe."[9]

The same system of Natural Law, born of that pure intelligence and perfect organizing power that orchestrates the totality of creation, also guides the functioning of human life. Health is the result of living in accord with these Laws of Nature.

The Five Elements of Nature

Everything in Nature—including the human physiology—unfolds from five basic elements, called *tanmatras*, which constitute the essence of the five senses. These subtle elements are the finest expression of material creation, and they are found at the "boundary" between consciousness or pure intelligence and matter. This picture of the finest strata of the objective world correlates with the profile of creation provided by quantum physics. Physicist John Hagelin, Ph.D., points out that physics has identified five major "spin types" that give rise to all of the elementary particles of physics, and that these spin types closely resemble the properties of the five tanmatras.

Five grosser elements, called *mahabhutas,* unfold from the tanmatras as their more concrete expression. The mahabhutas are the basic building blocks of the objective world. They structure the entire universe and everything in it—including your body and mind. From subtlest to most concrete, they are *akasha* (space), *vayu* (air), *tejas* or *agni* (fire), *apas* (water), and *prithivi* (earth).

It's easy to observe the five elements in Nature. For example, if you walk by a lake, you'll find yourself treading on the ground (earth), feeling the wind (air) in your hair and looking at the sun (fire) sparkling on the waves (water). As you move forward, your body moves through the subtlest element, space.

You are part of Nature, therefore these five elements are also the basic building blocks of your own body. The brain is composed of two-thirds water. Much of the body is composed of hollow space. Digestion breaks down food with heat (fire). The lungs breathe in air; and your bones are composed of the same chemicals and structure as the earth. The human body is an integral part of the body of Nature as a whole. For example, in the Vedic system, the same word (agni) refers both to the sun and to the digestive fire. This is one meaning of the expression, "As is the individual, so is the universe."

The Three Mind-Body Operators

To make it easier to analyze the human body, Maharishi Vedic Medicine reduces these five elements to three basic principles, called *doshas*: *Vata, Pitta,* and *Kapha.* These three doshas—Vata, Pitta, and Kapha—are composed of the five mahabhutas.

Five Elements and the Three Doshas

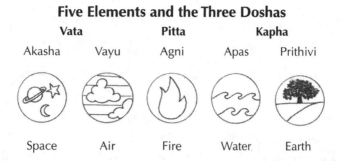

Vata		Pitta		Kapha
Akasha	Vayu	Agni	Apas	Prithivi
Space	Air	Fire	Water	Earth

The three doshas are the fundamental operators of every function in the mind and body. They each have different responsibilities. Vata governs motion. A thought moving through the mind, food moving down the digestive tract, blood moving through veins, breath being expelled from lungs—Vata governs all these movements.

Pitta governs heat, metabolism, and energy production. The conversion of food, air, and water into energy is controlled by Pitta dosha, as are hormonal cycles and functions. Kapha dosha controls physical structure and fluid balance. The formation of bones, muscles, and lymphatic systems are all in Kapha's realm.

Each of the three doshas has different qualities that appear in mind, body, and emotions. Vata is fast moving, quick, light, cold, minute, rough, dry. It is often called the king of the doshas, because the other doshas are inert without it. Pitta's qualities are hot, sharp, light, acidic and slightly oily. Kapha is heavy, oily, slow, cold, steady, solid and dull.

Different people have different proportions of the three doshas. Someone with a predominance of Vata will have a quick and lively mind and may walk fast. More Kapha might produce oily skin or strong muscles. Someone with a lot of Pitta in his body may digest food more quickly or feel overheated when he exercises.

The doshas are also found all around us in Nature. The seasons provide one obvious example. In the cool, wet spring, Kapha is more evident. In the hot summer, Pitta dosha dominates. Winter expresses the cold, dry, windy qualities of Vata.

A Detailed Picture of the Body's Functioning

The three doshas are present at every level of our mind-body system. Ayurvedic texts describe the different functions of the three doshas in complete detail. This section contains a brief overview of how the three doshas work.

Each of the three doshas has five subdoshas, which are located in different parts of the body. The subdivisions of Vata all relate to movement. The subdivisions of Pitta are concerned with digestion, heat, and metabolism. Those under Kapha are concerned with moistening and maintaining body structure.

The Qualities and Locations of the Three Doshas in Nature and Your Body

Vata: Moving, quick, light, cold, minute, rough, dry, leads the other doshas

Pitta: Hot, sharp, light, acidic, slightly oily, liquid, flowing

Kapha: Heavy, oily, slow, cold, steady solid, dull, soft, sweet, smooth

Locations of the Doshas in the Body

The doshas are found throughout the body. They reside in the body tissues and also in the organs formed by the tissues. They are more predominant in certain sites, or seats in the body.

Dosha	Chief Site	Secondary Sites
Vata	Large intestine	Waist, thighs, bones, ears, skin.
Pitta	Region around the navel	Stomach, duodenum, small intestine, liver, spleen, pancreas, lymph, blood, sweat, eye, and skin.
Kapha	Chest	Throat, head, pancreas, joints, stomach, fat, tongue, nose

---

The Five Subdoshas of Vata

Name and Meaning	Location	Function
Prana (vital breath)	Head, chest (including heart and respiratory organs), throat, tongue, mouth and nose	Breathing, sneezing, swallowing, belching; mental clarity; sensory perception, especially hearing and touch.
Udana (moving upward)	Throat, chest, navel	Speech, singing, swallowing; vitality and complexion.
Samana (moving evenly)	Umbilical region (stomach, intestines)	Fans the fire of appetite and digestion; stimulates enzyme production; moves food through the stomach and intestines.
Apana (moving downward)	Colon, rectum, bladder, thighs, groin	Elimination, menstruation, reproductive organs, navel, sexual discharge, delivery of fetus.
Vyana (moving in different directions; spreading)	All over the body, including circulatory and nervous systems	General movement of the body, extension and contraction, circulation of blood, also of lymph and sweat; sense of touch.

The Five Subdoshas of Pitta

Name and Meaning	Location	Function
Pachaka (to digest, to transform, to cook)	Small intestine (mainly duodenum); lower third of stomach	Digestion; maintaining the digestive fire through pancreatic, liver, and intestinal secretions.
Ranjaka (to color)	Liver, spleen	Regulates the blood chemistry and gives color to the blood.
Sadhaka (to achieve, to fulfill)	Heart	Desiring; fulfilling desires; intelligence, mental acuity, memory, enthusiasm, energy.
Alochaka (to see completely)	Visual system, including the eyes and visual cortex	Outer and inner vision.
Bhrajaka (to light, to shine)	Skin	Luster and shades of skin color; absorption through the skin.

The Five Subdoshas of Kapha

Name and Meaning	Location	Function
Kledaka (to moisten)	Stomach	Regulates initial phases of digestion, especially moistening the food.
Avalambaka (double supporting)	Chest, heart, lower back	Supports physical strength and stamina; regulates moisture in the lungs.
Bodhaka (to obtain knowledge)	Tongue, throat	Moistening the mouth; sense of taste; secretion of mucus in the mouth.
Tarpaka (pleasing nourishing)	Head, cerebrospinal fluid	Nourishes and lubricates organs of the head; nourishes the sensory and cognitive faculties and motor organs.
Shleshaka (to stick, bind, join)	Joints	Lubricates the joints; helps maintain structural integrity of the entire body.

Balanced Doshas Mean Perfect Health

When the three doshas are in balance, you enjoy perfect health. However, the doshas are constantly fluctuating and can easily lose their equilibrium. The normal qualities of the doshas then become exaggerated and create discomfort in mind, body, or emotions. If the imbalance continues to build, it leads to disease.

Balanced Vata creates mental alertness, normal elimination, sound sleep, strong immunity and a sense of exhilaration. If Vata is out of balance, it might produce dry or rough skin, insomnia, constipation, fatigue, tension headaches, intolerance of cold, low weight, anxiety and worry.

Signs of balanced Pitta include normal body heat and thirst, strong digestion, a shiny complexion, sharp intellect and contentment. Rashes, inflammatory skin diseases, peptic ulcers, heartburn, visual problems, excessive body heat or sweating, premature graying or baldness, and hostility and irritability are all signs that Pitta is out of balance.

When Kapha is normal, a person enjoys muscular strength, vitality and stamina, strong immunity, affection, generosity, courage, dignity, stability of mind and healthy joints. Imbalanced Kapha produces oily skin, slow digestion, sinus congestion, nasal allergies, asthma, cysts and other growths, and obesity.

You will learn more about the doshas in the next chapters, which investigate the causes of disease.

The Body Tissues

One important way that the three doshas express themselves is through body tissues, called *dhatus*, meaning "that which sustains." Ayurvedic texts identify seven body tissues.

The Seven Body Tissues

Rasa—plasma, the first product of digestion and metabolism

Rakta—blood, including hemoglobin

Mamsa—muscle tissue

Meda—fat tissue

Asthi—bone tissue

Majja—bone marrow, tissue of the nervous system

Shukra—reproductive tissues

The doshas govern the dhatus, and the dhatus make up the organs of the body. The Ayurvedic texts define disorder in the body as abnormality of the doshas and dhatus. Their equilibrium is equivalent to normality or health.

All the body tissues need to be balanced for the body to be healthy. An imbalance in any one of them can lead to disease. For example, multiple sclerosis indicates that there is an imbalance in *majja* dhatu, which includes the nervous system. An imbalance in *shukra* dhatu can result in infertility, and an imbalance in *rakta* dhatu causes anemia.

Malas

Healthy elimination is another important area related to balanced dhatus and doshas. It's commonly know that the human body eliminates impurities through the feces, urine and sweat. Looking more deeply, we find that the process of forming each of the dhatus produces normal waste products, called *malas*. If there is some blockage and one of these areas can't function normally, toxins and impurities accumulate, restricting the natural flow of intelligence and nourishment in the body. The body then gets thrown out of balance. When toxins accumulate, they mask the body's natural healing systems. That is why the removal of toxins and impurities is an important area of the Maharishi Vedic Approach to Health. This helps the body's natural elimination systems to function normally.

The Seven Tissues (Dhatus) and Their Normal Waste Products (Malas)

Dhatu	Mala
Rasa (plasma)	phlegm
Rakta (blood)	bile
Mamsa (muscle)	excreta from the outer openings (ears, eyes, mouth, nose, roots of hair)
Meda (fat)	sweat
Asthi (bone)	head and body hair, finger and toenails
Majja (bone marrow, nervous system)	oily substances in the eyes, skin, and feces
Shukra (reproductive)	no waste product

The subdoshas, dhatus, and malas together are the main components of the human body, and the body, mind, and consciousness together make up the total picture of health.

In this chapter, you have seen that the individual is an integral part of Nature. People suffering from chronic disorders often forget their connection to Nature and the entire cosmos, which is especially debilitating. The universe is vast and powerful, intricately engineered and orderly in its design. If you feel disconnected from the healing power of Nature, you can feel powerless indeed.

It is important to realize that even if you sometimes feel sick or powerless to heal yourself, you never lose the potential to change your condition from within. Consider this: DNA contains three trillion bits of information, and only one-and-a-half billion of those bits are necessary to govern the transformations of your human body. Since all the possible transformations in the universe are less than three trillion, your DNA not only manifests and manages your body, but also has enough potential information and organizing power to govern the entire universe, from the smallest particle to the largest galaxy. This is the potential you hold inside. You certainly have the power to overcome disease.

When you think of the miraculous intelligence that operates the mind-body—how many billions of neurons and cells and muscles must coordinate to enable you to walk, talk, think, breathe, or do the thousands of daily tasks that you take for granted—it is hard to believe that disease is possible at all.

Disease comes about only when some part of the body somehow loses connection with this perfectly functioning inner intelligence.

The next chapter explains how disease gets created from a disruption of the flow of the body's intelligence. Like stagnant pools of water that get cut off from the flow of the river, diseased areas of the body lose their communication with the source of life, consciousness. If the river starts to flood, those pools get swept away. When the flow of Nature's intelligence is restored to a diseased area, the disorder is washed away. All it takes is a flood of consciousness, a reconnection with the source of the body's healing and organizing intelligence, to eliminate illness. All it takes to remove darkness is switching on the light.

PART II
The Origin of Disease

The Origin of Disease

This section of the book explores etiology, the study of the causes of disease. Maharishi Vedic Medicine's viewpoint is refreshingly different from that of modern medicine. It locates one underlying cause for disease—the mind-body's disengagement from pure consciousness. Once this disconnection from Nature's intelligence and infinite organizing power is recognized as the primary cause of sickness, it can be treated successfully. Rather than concentrating on isolated symptoms, the Maharishi Vedic Approach to Health identifies and corrects the fundamental source of illness. This is what makes it so effective in treating chronic disease.

Chapter 4 examines the common origin of all sickness—a breakdown in the link between consciousness and the mind-body. Chapter 5 looks at the secondary causes of disease—mistakes in diet, lifestyle, and behavior.

How Disease Begins

"It is vital for the success of health care that the life of every individual is maintained in perfect alliance with Cosmic Life: that the health of the individual life is balanced and stable as the health of Cosmic Life, and the health of the nation is upheld by the perfect health of Cosmic Life." —*Maharishi Mahesh Yogi*[10]

Peggy, once an active businesswoman and writer, had been bed-bound for an entire year with symptoms that started as allergies, developed into asthma, and finally became a range of chronic problems. Extensive diagnostic tests revealed that she had hypothyroid/ Hashimoto syndrome, chronic allergies, chronic asthma verging on emphysema, chronic liver disease, chronic pancreatis, rheumatoid arthritis, depression, obesity, and cholesterol levels over 400. In addition, her doctor said she would need back surgery.

She couldn't eat anything except soup because her appetite had disappeared, yet she gained abnormal amounts of weight. Asthma made breathing difficult. Each day she took twelve to fourteen pills—including asthma medication, pain killers, migraine medicine, muscle relaxants, thyroid hormones, and sleeping pills—plus four or five asthma inhalers.

"At that point my mother told me, 'You've got to go somewhere for treatment because you are slowly dying,'" remembers Peggy. "I didn't have an immune system left."

Fortunately, Peggy made a decision to go to The Raj, an in-residence Maharishi Ayur-Veda Health center in Fairfield, Iowa, where she received a full range of therapies from Maharishi Vedic Medicine. "When I finished my eight days there I had my energy back," she says. "I went back to all my specialists and had the same diagnostic tests, and they told me that suddenly I no longer had asthma, not a trace. There were no imbalances in the blood, no chronic liver problems, no pancreatic problems. My thyroid is absolutely normal, and my cholesterol level is now down to 200. The rheumatoid arthritis is gone, and I no longer need back surgery."

Peggy still has to take medication for her thyroid and migraines, but otherwise she sticks to Maharishi Ayur-Veda™ herbal compounds to strengthen her liver and pancreas. She also follows a daily routine and diet prescribed for her at the The Raj.

Besides curing her chronic illnesses, Peggy feels that her new knowledge of Maharishi Vedic Medicine has changed her whole life. "When I was sick, I'd look at myself in the mirror and think, 'Who is this old lady?'" says Peggy. "Now I feel like I'm twenty-five. My skin is radiant and I look younger than I did before. Without even trying I lost twenty to thirty pounds right from the start, and have now lost fifty pounds. There are all these side benefits to following these natural therapies. I feel consciousness moving through me now." As Peggy likes to say, she arrived in a wheelchair and she left dancing.

While few people have as many different diseases as Peggy, chronic disease is by nature complicated and usually involves many organs and systems. It affects the mind, body, and emotions. Disease starts long before it manifests as a symptom. By the time symptoms such as asthma, arthritis, heart disease, or liver disease become a day-to-day reality, many years of imbalance have already passed.

In my practice, I have seen over and over again that trying to treat only the symptoms of a disorder, or even just trying to treat the organ systems involved—for example, the digestive system or the reproductive system—does not produce lasting results. The beauty and simplicity of Maharishi Vedic Medicine lies in its understanding that an underlying source of imbalance creates these myriad symptoms and signs of illness. Peggy's case dramatically illustrates this point: All her symptoms disappeared once the origin of the disease was eliminated.

By having a clearer understanding of the basis of disease, it becomes much easier to treat the patient in a holistic fashion. In this context, treatment of the patient as a whole is a necessity and eradicating the root cause is a must. Maharishi Vedic Medicine uses a different understanding of the etiology (cause) and pathology (progression) of disease. Until you understand how disorders both start and build, you cannot understand how to undo them.

How Disease Starts

The modern view of disease does not consider the underlying field of Nature's intelligence, which operates all the myriad cells of the body. Just as the vast ocean is hidden under the waves at the surface, so the vast, silent field of Nature's intelligence, or pure consciousness, is hidden beneath the endless activity of human life. The physical body is merely one expression of it.

At the moment when any part of the body gets disconnected from its basis in unbounded intelligence, disease begins. If you can reestablish the connection with that infinite field of energy, perfect orderliness, and bliss, then you can restore balance to the physiology.

The purpose of Maharishi Vedic Medicine is to reestablish the connection between the body and its inner intelligence. This inner intelligence, or pure consciousness, is so intimately linked with the body that the two are essentially one—the body *is* intelligence, consciousness itself. As Peggy experienced, all of the approaches of Maharishi Vedic Medicine reestablish the link with this field of inner intelligence and bring balance to every cell in the body.

Maharishi Vedic Medicine views sickness as caused by lack of complete knowledge. If people don't know or fully experience themselves as the infinite field of happiness, orderliness, power, and balance that is the Veda, then they fall sick. The body's inner intelligence never changes. It is always radiating health. However, just as a cloud can cover the sun, sometimes the inner intelligence is as if shadowed. You lose your awareness of it, lose your ability to know it as your own essential nature. When the relationship between the body and its source of perfect orderliness and organizing power gets weakened or lost, illness starts.

The one major cause of disease in the human body, then, is the inability to experience your fundamental nature, who you really are. The loss of the body's partnership with its internal source of intelligence has a special name in Maharishi Vedic Medicine: *pragya-aparadh*—"the mistake of the intellect."

The Mistake of the Intellect

Physicians trained in Maharishi Vedic Medicine understand the influence of toxins as well as imbalances in the body tissues and functions. They also know the role of bacteria or viruses in generating disease. However, they look first at the primary cause of illness, pragya-aparadh. In simple terms, this "mistake of the intellect" means that the mind loses its connection to its source, forgets its true identity with the total potential of Natural Law, the field of wholeness within. This loss of memory causes the person to violate the Laws of Nature in thought, speech, and action.

The enlightened individual, by definition, is fully united with his infinite nature and therefore enjoys perfect health. Every thought and action for this person is in tune with the total potential of Natural Law, and he therefore does not make mistakes. In other words, he does not violate Natural Law and damage himself, other individuals, or his environment. All that he does supports life as a whole. Such person is always connected with his source. Every cell in his body is flooded with the light of inner intelligence, and consequently, he never falls sick.

You are already designed to live in harmony with the Laws of Nature that govern the beautiful universe of which you are a part. You are designed to enjoy unbounded energy, perfect orderliness, and perfect health. It is only when you get disconnected from the infinite reservoir of wholeness within that ill health and suffering begin.

Forgetting That You Are Pure Consciousness

You could think of your awareness as a river. As the river flows, it goes through hills, dales, deserts, towns, and villages. It meets people and animals, nourishing all the areas around it. But it doesn't become the things that it passes—it remains the river. In the same way, you pass through enormous changes in human experience everyday. Your experience overwhelming happiness one moment and great challenges the next. Whatever the circumstances, you need to remain your true self. That's what Maharishi Vedic Medicine does—it connects you back to the unified level of the Self in the midst of the diversity of life. It anchors you to the silent depth of the ocean while the waves move on the surface.

All of the therapies of Maharishi Vedic Medicine help enliven the source of pure silence, energy, and intelligence within. When you are able to maintain pure awareness, restful alertness, twenty-four hours a day, while sleeping, dreaming, and waking, then pragya-aparadh will be gone. The bliss of pure consciousness will be enjoyed continuously in daily life. No experience, no matter how pleasurable or painful, will overshadow that bliss.

Pragya-aparadh is a state in which you do not remember that you are unbounded, all-knowing consciousness. Instead, you identify with the objects of your perception: your body, job, the environment, even disease. The mind is like a mirror, whose nature is to reflect objects. What then is the essential nature of the mirror? How can the mirror's nature be known if it is always covered by the objects it reflects? What if you could remove all the objects of perception, all the objects of the senses that cover or overshadow the mind's essential nature, pure awareness? This is what happens during the Transcendental Meditation technique. The Self is left alone by itself to experience its true reality, unbounded consciousness. Pure consciousness is a field of unlimited fullness and potential, an infinite continuum of wholeness, perfect orderliness, bliss, and harmony. When the mind is completely and permanently unified with pure consciousness, it never again gets lost in external circumstances or objects. You never again identify with boundaries or limited qualities of any kind. You never think: "I am this body," or "I am this sickness."

Pragya-aparadh and the
Three-in-One Structure of Consciousness

The essential feature of pure consciousness is awareness, or pure "knowingness," which gives it the quality of being aware of its own existence. While remaining absolutely whole and unified, consciousness, knowing itself, generates a threefold structure— knower, process of knowing, and object of knowledge or, (*rishi, devata*, and *chhandas*). This division is, however, purely virtual or conceptual. Consciousness is in reality all three—the knower, known, and the link between them.

Modern physics explains that the mathematical structure of the unified field is the blueprint for creation. Similarly, the three-in-one fabric of consciousness provides a kind of architectural foundation for the universe. As consciousness expresses itself as the manifest, physical creation—as it precipitates into matter— this three-in-one quality is found everywhere and in everything. It is an unchanging relationship that provides the formula for all change and orderliness in an ever-evolving universe. In the structure of the human physiology, it appears as the three doshas— Vata, Pitta, and Kapha.

In a state of perfect health, these three values are experienced in their true unity, called *samhita*. Pragya-aparadh occurs when the intellect, the discriminating value of consciousness, loses its connection to wholeness. It starts to identify with the endless diversity of life, the vast field of objective creation, rather than with the fundamental unity of life in which subject and object are one. When the knower gets lost in the world of objects due to the mistake of his intellect, he is cut off from the field of infinite orderliness that orchestrates every structure and function of his mind-body. This is the primary cause of disease.

Rishi, devata, and chhandas represent the world as you experience it through the senses. Samhita, the unified state of rishi, devata, and chhandas, is like the unseen sap underlying all the different parts of a tree. The colorless sap nourishes the entire tree, and every leaf and cell of the tree is connected to it. Without the sap, the tree would die. Our whole mind-body is an expression of samhita. It supports everything that you are and everything that you do. Though you cannot see it, you would have no life, no existence, without it.

If an individual loses his connection to samhita—that is, begins to perceive himself and his world as diversified, separate parts, disconnected from wholeness, then he is suffering from pragya-aparadh. Pragya-aparadh is the experience of the diversity of creation at the expense of unity—identification with the parts, rather than the underlying wholeness.

This is the first step of disease. Consciousness keeps every part of the body and mind running in health and harmony. If you forget your true nature, you lose access to the field of infinite orderliness, the home of all the Laws of Nature, which is meant to guide every step and manifestation of life to its fulfillment. You run the risk of violating Natural Law in your thoughts and actions. These violations generate disease.

How Pragya-aparadh Leads to Disease

Natural Law is responsible for the ordering and evolution of every facet of the created universe. A violation of Natural Law

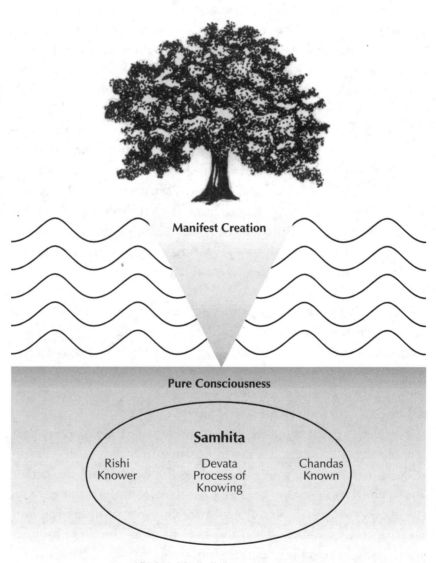

Manifest Creation

Pure Consciousness

Samhita

Rishi	Devata	Chandas
Knower	Process of	Known
	Knowing	

Unified Field of all the Laws of Nature

produces disorder in bodily communication and function, which in turn becomes sickness. For health, every part must be connected to the common source. When there is disorder, the connection gets muddled. It creates a shadow, and as the shadow thickens, disorder grows. It is like the game of telephone you may have played as a child. The first person whispers a sentence into the second person's ear, who whispers it into the third person's ear, and so on. Each time it is whispered, the sentence gets more confused. By the time the sentence travels around the circle, it is completely distorted. In the same way, as the connection of inner intelligence to the tissues diminishes, the cells gradually lose their perfect functioning.

When the body is no longer connected to its inner intelligence, the experience of the Self is shadowed. Alertness is shadowed and thinking becomes disorderly. As the shadow thickens, inner communication with the Self becomes increasingly difficult. Like the telephone game, disorder gets magnified with each generation of faulty communication.

As intelligence begins to bypass the affected tissues, the tissue cells start to freeze. Like a flower cut off from its nourishing sap, the moment that cells lose their link with samhita, they become frozen in time. Once frozen, the cells forget how to function according to their original, perfect, immortal blueprint. Having lost connection with the body's governing intelligence, the cells and tissues start to function out of synchrony with the body as a whole.

The solution to disease is to create health. All forty approaches of Maharishi Vedic Medicine create the desired result. They dissolve pragya-aparadh and structure enlightenment. Sickness disappears as an automatic byproduct.

I once heard a story about a saint. He said, "When I was young I tried to change the whole world. When I was middle-aged, I thought, 'This will never work. Let me just change the friends and relatives around me.' In old age it dawned on me that the only person I can change is myself." You can make the most profound and lasting changes within yourself by basing all transformations on your reconnection to the source of life within. When you change from that level, you change not only yourself but also everything around you.

How Pragya-aparadh Leads to
Mistakes in Thought, Speech and Action

Losing the memory of your real nature can cause you to make mistakes in many different areas of life. When you don't know who you really are, you also forget your intimacy with nature and with the universe as a whole. You can no longer feel the influence of our environment, neither near or far—the sun, moon, or planets. It all comes back to pragya-aparadh. Losing your intimacy with consciousness leads to mistakes in thought and behavior, which breeds disease.

Maharishi Vedic Medicine provides the knowledge and techniques to bring back the fullest experience of your unlimited, blissful nature. The Transcendental Meditation technique restores the experience of pure consciousness. All forty treatment modalities, including diet and lifestyle recommendations suited to each individual constitution, reestablish balance in the mind-body and enliven Nature's healing intelligence. When you overcome pragya-aparadh, you are spontaneously attracted to a healthy daily routine and diet.

Like a kite on a string, most of us need to maintain our connection to the source of life even while we are pulling away from it. Every business must be supported by the bank, by sufficient capital resources. If you lose access to your inner bank, you get tired. Your thinking gets disorderly and you start to make poor choices in diet and lifestyle as well as many other areas of life. If you continue to act in ways that violate Natural Law, toxins and free radicals accumulate, and eventually a disease develops. In the next chapter, you will learn about the different ways that mistakes in diet, behavior, and speech can produce disease.

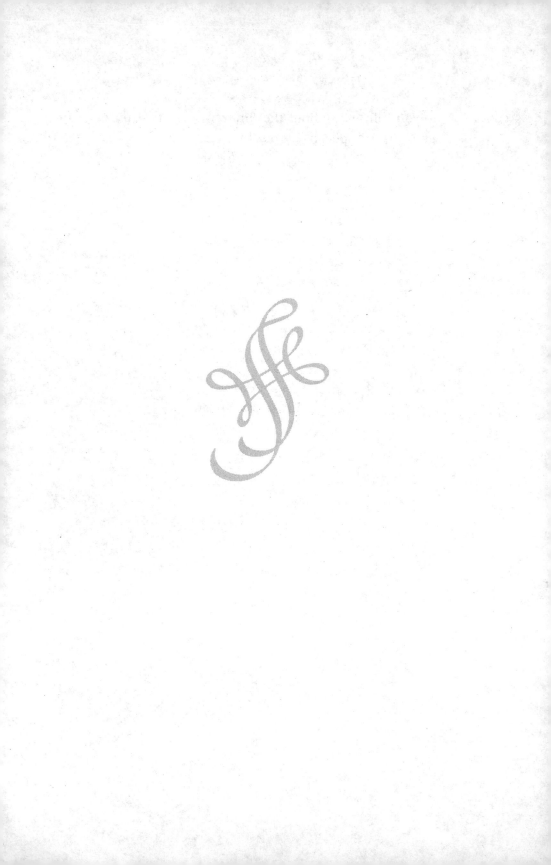

CHAPTER 5

Behavior, Diet, Doshas and Disease

"Ill health is fundamentally due to violation of Natural Law caused by lack of knowledge of Natural Law. Lack of knowledge of Natural Law weakens the individual and creates stress in society."

—*Maharishi Mahesh Yogi*[11]

Paul, a psychotherapist, started having sinus problems in his late 20s. They became more and more severe, and eventually developed into a chronic inflammation of the nasal and sinus passages. Sinus polyps (growths) blocked his breathing and sense of smell. These had to be periodically removed by surgery. By the time he was 47, asthma set in, making his breathing so difficult that he had to take Prednisone® and medicated sprays.

When he came to my office three years ago, he had already tried some alternative approaches without success. However, after Paul used a number of procedures from Maharishi Vedic Medicine—including dietary changes, herbal supplements, internal purification treatments, and purification therapies for the nasal passages—Paul was able to break the cycle of surgery.

"The pattern had gotten to the point that every two years I was developing a new polyp," he says. "The two-year mark has come and gone and I'm not in a lot of trouble. I'm holding my own." Paul has his polyp tissue monitored closely, and although some tissue remains, it's not out of control.

In addition, Paul has greatly reduced his use of nasal sprays and decongestants, and the asthma has improved dramatically. He only occasionally has bouts where he has to use the Prednisone and sprays for a few days.

"I feel like I'm healing," he says. "I'm a lot healthier now than I was three years ago. My goal is to not need any medication, and now I think that's possible."

He says that the Transcendental Meditation technique helps him stay more grounded. "I'm emotionally more stable now. When you live with a chronic illness, it affects every aspect of your life. If you decrease your suffering, it frees up a lot of energy to expend in other ways. Rather than just trying to get through the day and deal with symptoms, now my relationships, my work, everything has improved."

In the third chapter we saw that the mistake of the intellect—its identification with objects of perception rather than its source in consciousness—is the primary cause of disease. However, many secondary causes, which are the direct result of this fundamental error, can also cause disease. When the mind-body loses access to its governing intelligence, the home of all the Laws of Nature, you may begin to think and act in ways that contradict or violate Natural Law in any area of life. These breaches of Natural Law may include improper diet, an unhealthy daily routine, flaws in sensory perception or exposing the senses to damaging input, mental errors, mistakes in speech and action, and mistakes related to time or the seasons.

Errors That Cause Disease

The *Charaka Samhita*, an age-old textbook used by Maharishi Vedic Medicine, says, "Due to pragya-aparadh, the ignorant indulge in unwholesome gratification of the five senses, suppression of natural urges, exposure to strain beyond their capacity and adoption of such regimes as bring only temporary happiness. But the wise do not indulge in them because of their clarity of vision."[12]

Errors made in four major areas of life constitute the main sources of illness:

1. Mind, speech, and behavior
2. Sensory perception
3. Diet
4. Time (seasonal and daily routines, etc.)

The *Charaka Samhita* states that the "causes of disease relating to both mind and body are wrong usage, nonusage, and excessive usage of time, mental faculties, and objects of the sense organs. Balanced use of time, mental faculties, and sense organs is the cause of happiness."[13]

The disease process begins whenever there is excessive use, nonuse, or wrong use of the elements in any one of the four main arenas of experience. For example, if you habitually eat too much, or too little, or eat the wrong foods for your constitution, you may be creating imbalance or sickness. Paul, for instance, had developed an imbalance through his diet and lifestyle that accumulated over time.

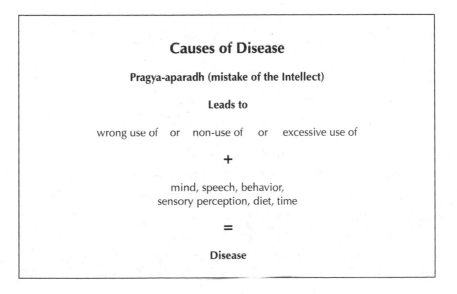

Causes of Disease

Pragya-aparadh (mistake of the Intellect)

Leads to

wrong use of   or   non-use of   or   excessive use of

+

mind, speech, behavior,
sensory perception, diet, time

=

Disease

How Mind, Speech and Behavior Can Cause Disease

What you think, say and do each day can have positive or negative effects on your health. Excessive or insufficient use as well as wrong use of thought, speech or action can lead to disease. For example, if a person does too much mental work—too much thinking or calculating for long periods of time—it can cause an imbalance. On the other hand, not using the mind at all can also be detrimental to health.

Negative emotions such as fear, grief, anger, greed, jealousy, passion, and finding fault with others can actually result in sickness. Such emotions have an effect on the entire body, but the weakest areas will react more strongly to the stress factors. For example, if someone already has a Pitta imbalance, experiencing excessive anger, excitement or irritation can contribute to the development of hypertension or gastric ulcers. Fear, grief or anxiety, on the other hand, could trigger an asthma attack.

Doshas and Negative Emotions		
Vata	*Pitta*	*Kapha*
Fear	Anger	Passion
Grief	Excitement	Greed
Anxiety	Irritation	Jealousy
Stress	Hyperacidity	Stress
	Hypertension	

Speaking too much or for long periods of time can produce hoarseness, coughs and other disorders localized in the throat. Speech that is quarrelsome, harsh, irrelevant, impolite, abusive, or that focuses on others' faults can generate illness.

Improper exercise, overexercise (professional football players have an average life span of fifty-six years), excessive sexual activity, or too much traveling can weaken health. On the other hand, a lack of exercise can be extremely debilitating and can lead to a wide range of disorders.

Actions that endanger or weaken life, such as alcohol or drug use, inhalation of polluted air, or exposure to fire or radiation, may also result in ill health.

Suppressing natural urges such as sneezing, urination or bowel movement is an important cause of disease. The body speaks to you through its natural urges. If you ignore these signals, you interfere with the threshold of communication in that area, and the muscles and nerves begin to lose their ability to react appropriately. If you repeatedly interfere, the organs lose the strength they need to function at the proper time in response to the proper signal. Once the sequence is lost, the muscles and nerves respond in a confused way. In addition, toxins start to build up if the body cannot remove waste properly. Headaches, including migranes, sinus problems, urinary problems, constipation, diarrhea and irritable bowel syndrome can result from suppressing the impulse to sneeze, urinate or move the bowels.

The Three Mental Qualities

The mind (*manas*) plays a significant role in the creation of health or disease, because the mind's disposition can either strengthen or weaken the function of the body's systems. The Vedic texts outline three different mental qualities, or ways in which the mind operates. These are called *gunas—rajas, sattva* and *tamas*—and they are related to the physical doshas (Vata, Pitta, and Kapha) described in Chapter 2. The influence of the gunas is all-pervasive. They govern the processes of creation, destruction and maintenance throughout the universe.

Sattva

Sattva is said to be pure, illuminating, beneficial. A sattvic mind is calm, benevolent, creative, imaginative, inspired. It is responsive to knowledge, capable of gaining correct knowledge through the senses and has the desire for knowledge. Sattva is ideal for the maintaining of health.

Rajas

Rajas produces action. It is expressed in mental dynamism, thinking, analyzing, discriminating and focusing. Rajas is unsteady, constantly moving, quick, and strong. When rajas is out of balance, the mind becomes unstable, irritable and reactive. It develops passion, attachment, desire, hatred, worry, grief, fear, jealousy, pride and many other unhealthy emotions. It is incapable of understanding and responding to circumstances in a healthy or appropriate way.

Tamas

Tamas is found in the ability to synthesize, draw conclusions, memorize, and establish thoughts and ideas. It finishes whatever is created by sattva and actualized or implemented by rajas. When it is out of balance, tamas is static, slow, inhibiting and obstructing. The mind becomes slow to understand and react and incapable of adapting suitably to situations. It develops ignorance, worry, delusion and other negative emotions.

Every physical body is composed of the same cells, organs, and tissues, yet you react to experience in many different ways. Your response to experience originates in the mind. The nature of the response depends on the balance of the gunas. It also directly affects your body and your health. Sattva is always beneficial for the mind, no matter how much it increases. You cannot have too much sattva—it predictably yields health and balance. Only the decrease of sattva can lead to disease.

Rajas and tamas are also fundamental players in the mind's functioning. However, if you lose the natural balance of the gunas through excessive rajas or tamas, ill health is a likely result. When the influence of rajas or tamas in the mind becomes too great, the mind loses its faculty of discrimination and memory. You cannot make healthy choices and you cannot understand or react to situations correctly. For example, too much rajas or tamas inevitably produces poor decisions about food and lifestyle. These in turn can cause abnormal doshas and disease.

Relationship of Three Gunas and Three Doshas				
Samhita	Rishi	Knower	Sattva	Vata
	Devata	Knowing	Rajas	Pitta
	Chhandas	Known	Tamas	Kapha

Qualities of Balanced Gunas

Sattva: Light, illuminating, clear, happy; origination of thoughts and ideas.

Rajas: Mentally dynamic, analytical, discriminating, focused, organized, active, in motion.

Tamas: Synthesizing, summarizing, memorizing; established thoughts and ideas.

Qualities of Imbalanced Gunas

Sattva: Decreased sattva can lead to disease.

Rajas: Irritable, quick to react, passionate, attached; prone to hatred, worry, grief, fear, jealousy, pride, and other unhealthy emotions.

Tamas: Slow to understand and react, incapable of suitable adaption to life's situations; prone to ignorance, worry, delusion, and other negative emotions.

When an individual's awareness is established in pure consciousness, his mind and body are fully connected to and totally governed by that infinite intelligence. In this state, the reference point for all physiological changes, whether they are due to the body's natural requirements or environmental demands, is the unchanging, absolutely stable field of pure Being. The whole mind-body system maintains coherent functioning no matter what the challenge, and the individual remains healthy irrespective of the demands and difficulties of life.

When the individual is disconnected from Nature's intelligence, the brain loses its capacity for coherent functioning and the mind-body connection becomes distorted. The result is a disruption and weakening of at least part of the physiology, which can in turn produce disease.

As long as sattva, rajas, and tamas are balanced, they support the connections among every part of the physiology with its underlying wholeness in consciousness. When their natural balance is not maintained—when the influence of tamas or rajas starts to predominate—the link with consciousness, the infinite intelligence that orchestrates all the activity in the mind-body, is clouded. The individual's choices about food and lifestyle start to be overshadowed by rajas or tamas. Emotions and behavior then start to reflect excessive rajas or tamas. Confused or destructive diet and lifestyle choices or behaviors will in turn produce imbalance in the doshas. This is how the quality of the mind starts affecting the body and the doshas.

Each of the forty approaches of Maharishi Vedic Medicine supports the growth and maintenance of sattva in the mind. One of the main results of the Transcendental Meditation technique in particular is that the individual spontaneously makes decisions about food, daily routine and behavior that create health or, you could say, makes decisions that are in tune with Natural Law. The key word is *spontaneously*. When a person *really wants* to eat good food and be on a healthy routine and is automatically, even instinctively, attracted to life-supporting choices, that is when healing really begins. All my patients tell me that they started to get well when there was a change in their perception, and in their quality of thinking. They changed how they thought about themselves, their illnesses and their lifestyles.

Diet, Daily Routine, and Health

In Maharishi Vedic Medicine, diet is one of the pillars of health. Many times even serious diseases start to turn around when someone begins to eat properly. Remember that the three gunas pervade creation, and are therefore found in every kind of food in different proportions. Consequently, the food you eat influences your mind-set.

Foods that have sattva, rajas and tamas in the right proportions are good for everyone. They create a light, blissful feeling in the mind and body. Foods with too much tamas can make the mind dull and prone to making mistakes. Excessive tamas can also cause frustration or depression, because it is difficult to fulfill your desires or maintain your responsibilities when the mind is sluggish. Foods with an imbalance of rajas can create strong emotions and cause too much excitation in the mind. Foods that are primarily sattvic produce mental clarity and exhilaration and are easily digested by the body.

All the dietary recommendations of Maharishi Vedic Medicine support health by promoting sattva. However, Maharishi Vedic Medicine recognizes the uniqueness of every individual. Each person has specific dietary needs. The many ways in which the three doshas—Vata, Pitta, and Kapha—combine in the human physiology produce a broad range of possibilities in each person's constitutional makeup. Like all physicians trained in Maharishi Vedic Medicine, after I diagnose people I give them a precise diet based on their particular doshic qualities and imbalances.

In many, many cases, just eating the suitable foods can have a remarkable effect in turning around disease. Paul, for example, was suffering from an underlying Kapha imbalance. This imbalance accumulated during his early years, and later erupted into his sinus problems and asthma. By altering his diet, he was able to reduce Kapha dosha and bring his entire body back into equilibrium.

Health and the Five Senses of Perception

You've probably heard the expression, "You are what you eat." Most people have a working understanding of how they take food from the environment and convert it into the nutrients that maintain their bodies. However, what most people don't know is that you also metabolize your environment with your senses.

Your sense organs take in information from the world around you that nourishes your body. If, however, a sensory stimulus is too strong, it can be harmful and can even create disease. On the other hand, if one of the sense organs is not stimulated at all, this can also be harmful. Sensory input that is distorted or unnatural is a third potential source of illness.

The Ayurvedic texts offer examples of this phenomenon:

Sight

Seeing too bright a light for long periods of time or remaining in very dim light or darkness can be detrimental. Sensitive or weak eyes, photophobia or night blindness can result. Seeing anything that is frightening, unusual, annoying, emotional, unnatural, or terrifying could generate disease.

Hearing

Loud, high-pitched sounds, too little sound, or a total lack of it are harmful to the sense of hearing. Harsh or terrifying words, words that convey loss of friends, relatives or money, or news of accidents or crimes can also trigger illness or cause hearing disorders, ringing in the ears, reduction in hearing ability, and ear pain.

Touch

Potentially harmful influences include touching very hot or

cold substances, excessive bathing or oil massages, no bath at all, or the complete lack of tactile experience. Research on abandoned infants who have not been caressed and touched lovingly by their parents shows dramatically how the emotions and physiology can be disturbed by lack of touch. In fact, babies who are not touched cannot survive, even if they are fed. Improper clothing or posture, contact with unclean objects, assault, invasion by worms, insects, and bacteria, and exposure to chemicals or pollutants can all damage health. Potential consequences include skin diseases, allergies, and hypersensitivity to hot, cold, or specific textures.

Taste

Misuse of the sense of taste can result in food allergies and loss of the ability to taste.

Smell

When the sense of smell is overwhelmed, misused, underused, or not used at all, disorders such as a decrease in the sense of smell or odor-related allergies can develop. Smelling toxins such as cigarette smoke, chemical vapors, or polluted air can weaken the senses and damage the body.

The Influence of Time

A fascinating area of Maharishi Vedic Medicine measures the influence of the cycles of the earth revolving around the sun (the four seasons) and the earth revolving on its axis (the daily rising and setting of the sun). These cycles produce obvious changes in your mind and body, and directly affect health.

Different doshas predominate during different seasons and different times of day. When they start accumulating in the body, they hold the potential for disease if that buildup is not addressed through adjustments in diet and daily routine. Most cultures tend to counteract the effects of the seasons with changes in their diet and lifestyles. You naturally eat heavier, warmer foods to counteract the light, cold, windy effects of Vata dosha in the winter. You tend to eat lighter, cooler foods in the hot, Pitta-dominant summer season. Everything slows down in summer, as you try to stay cool.

These cycles are thought of as external influences, because they are found in the environment around you and influence you from the outside. Other cycles of time influence you internally, such as the cycles of life. Throughout life, Vata, Pitta, and Kapha govern the three major periods in human development. Kapha is predominant when the bones, muscles, and structure of the body are being formed in childhood. Pitta predominates in middle age, when most people are extremely active, vital, and taking command of their lives. Vata takes over in old age, increasing vulnerablity to problems such as insomnia, dry skin, and weakness. To maintain balance and health throughout life, Maharishi Vedic Medicine prescribes foods and behavioral routines that take these influences into account.

Vata Season
Late Autumn to Early Winter

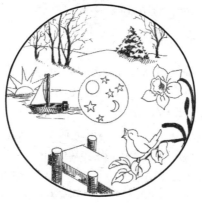

Pitta Season
Summer through
Early Autumn

Kapha Season
Spring through
Early Summer

The Maharishi Vedic Medicine physician also takes other internal cycles into account when he or she prescribes herbal compounds. There is an optimum time for different substances to interact with the body. The body's internal intelligence will respond differently to the intelligence contained in an herb at different points in the day. Some herbs work better in the morning, some before a meal, some after a meal, and so forth. Timing is always taken into account when Maharishi Ayur-Veda herbal preparations are prescribed.

Cycles of Digestion and Doshic Dominance

Kapha—first hour after eating
Pitta—second hour after eating
Vata—third hour after eating

In Western medicine, the influence of time has been studied in recent years as chronobiology. Research shows that the same pill you take at seven in the morning has a different effect later in the day. Recent studies also show that the biological clock of a young

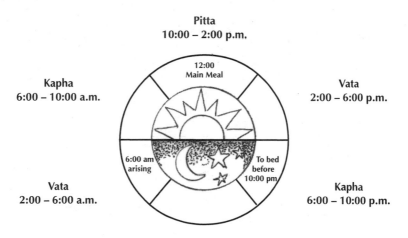

Pitta
10:00 – 2:00 p.m.

Kapha
6:00 – 10:00 a.m.

12:00
Main Meal

Vata
2:00 – 6:00 p.m.

6:00 am
arising

To bed
before
10:00 pm

Vata
2:00 – 6:00 a.m.

Kapha
6:00 – 10:00 p.m.

Pitta
10:00 – 2:00 a.m.

person is set differently than that of an older person. Furthermore, there is a set time or progression of disease.

The next chapters will clarify your understanding of how the mistakes of diet, behavior, thought, speech, action, use of the senses, and timing set in motion the series of transformations that take place when a healthy person becomes sick.

PART III
The Development of Disease

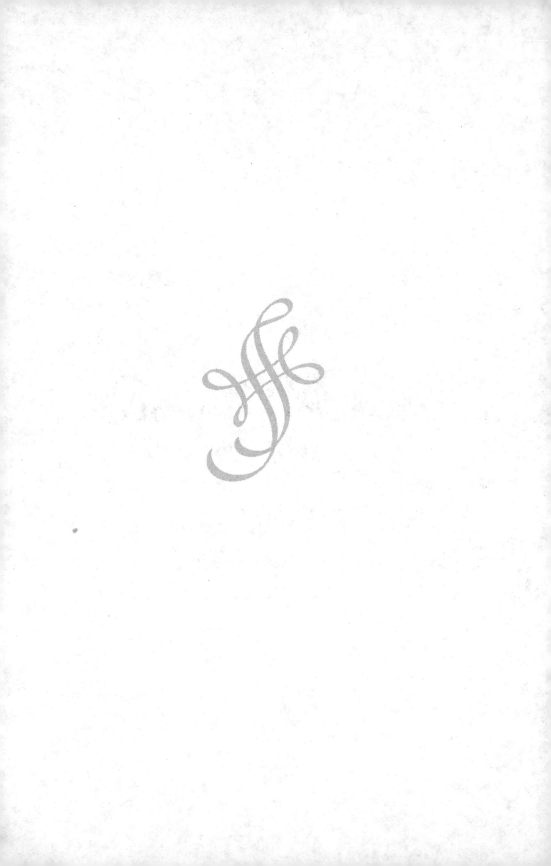

The Development of Disease

The last two chapters explored the origins of disease. You saw how the seed of disease is sown when pragya-aparadh disconnects you from the blueprint of intelligence that orchestrates the innumerable physiological activities of the human body. In this section, you will learn how disease progresses from preclinical imbalances in the body to vague feelings of discomfort before it eventually appears as full-blown symptoms. As you will see, Maharishi Vedic Medicine approaches the etiology of disease in a unique and comprehensive way. It gives invaluable insights into how disease develops over time if subtle physiological imbalances are allowed to take root and spread. When you truly understand this process, the steps of treatment and prevention follow naturally.

The key point in understanding the emergence of disease is the recognition that it is a long-term process, involving numerous changes in both body and mind. The following chapters outline all the facets of this development—from the first appearance of imbalances to disruption of digestion to distortion of body tissues and obstruction of the channels of circulation. Chapter 6 looks at how the disease process originates with the spread of imbalances to the bodily tissues. Chapter 7 examines the considerable role that weak digestion—and the resulting toxins and impurities— play in the development of disease. Chapter 8 focuses on what happens when the body's many channels of circulation get obstructed—another important step in the progression of disease. Chapter 9 describes how all these factors together form the six stages of disease that occur during the development of any illness. The stage of disease in which full-blown symptoms emerge, and which modern medicine generally considers to be the starting point of disease, corresponds to the *fourth* stage in the Ayurvedic model of the development of disease.

This section ends with Chapter 10, which presents case studies of two patients who suffered from asthma and arthritis. Their stories give a vivid example of the cause and progression of disease and how powerfully disease can be addressed using the techniques of Maharishi Vedic Medicine.

CHAPTER 6

From Doshas to Tissues—
The Spread of Imbalance

"It is in the interest of everyone, healthy or otherwise,
to own this knowledge of the total range of health—
from individual to cosmic—to maintain balance in life,
the basis of good health.

It should be understood that anything that is helpful
for maintenance of balance is also helpful to stop the
growth of imbalance...."   —*Maharishi Mahesh Yogi*[14]

By now you have a greater understanding of the physiological
imbalances that plant the first seeds of disease. How do these first
seeds of disease sprout and grow into full-blown symptoms, such
as arthritis, asthma or ulcers? The common understanding is that
disease develops in a certain part of the body—arthritis develops
in the joints, asthma in the lungs, and ulcers in the stomach. But
in actuality, the outbreak of disease in a specific area is just the expression of a far more pervasive process.

This process can be understood on many different levels. At
the deepest level, it means that the body has become disconnected from its source of wholeness—you are no longer fully attuned to that perfect cosmic blueprint, the infinite intelligence
that organizes and implements all bodily functions. This process
can also be conceived of in terms of the three doshas. Remember
from Chapter 3 that the three doshas—the three transformational principles that govern all the functions of the mind-body—

must be kept in balance to maintain ideal health. This chapter explains how doshic imbalances can migrate to the body tissues and cause disruption and disease.

Rx for Health: Balanced Doshas

The doshas are a vital part of physiological functioning. Together they govern the myriad processes that constitute the dynamic reality of the body. Each dosha regulates many aspects of the mind-body system, yet doshic functions can be summarized in three basic principles. Vata represents the element of air and controls any form of *movement* in the body. It governs blood circulation, the passage of food through the digestive tract, the breathing process, the movement of nerve impulses, energy, and so on. Pitta represents fire. It governs metabolism and biochemical processes, such as digestion, appetite and thirst. It also governs sight, heat, luster and complexion. It is responsible for the transformation of food, air and water into the building blocks of the physiology. Kapha represents the principle of structure and governs the formation of tissues, muscles, bones and sinews. Kapha functions include lubrication, binding, connection of the muscles and skin around the joints, healing and immunity.

When you enjoy perfect health, the mental and physical functions administered by each dosha are working properly. The doshas are in balance. That is, they are present in the body in the proper proportion, they exhibit the proper qualities, and they perform their prescribed functions.

The first phase of the disease process begins when the performance of one or more doshas is disturbed. If the imbalance is not addressed at this early stage, the disturbed or "aggravated" dosha can spread imbalance throughout the body, creating disease and destroying bodily tissues. By learning how to work with, instead of against, the operation of the doshas, you can prevent and even eliminate imbalances.

By diagnosing the doshic imbalances underlying a specific disease, a physician trained in Maharishi Vedic Medicine often is able to address problems that don't respond to the therapies of Western medicine. One of my patients, 49-year-old Amy, offers a case in point. She was plagued by frequent urinary tract infections for two years. Her other doctors had treated her with antibiotics, and in addition she had tried several natural therapies before she came to me. However, in spite of her best efforts, the treatments provided only marginal relief. Even worse, her immune system was so weakened by the recurrent antibiotic treatments that she had become stuck in a debilitating vicious circle. With the help of antibiotics, she would recover from one infection only to fall prey to another a few weeks later. The recurring infections left her feeling depleted and run down. When she came to me, she was still suffering from urinary tract infections, and also was complaining of serious fatigue, lack of appetite and painful backaches.

I immediately put Amy on a treatment program that would strengthen her immune system and would also address the doshic imbalances that caused the urinary infections. Urinary tract infections are often caused by a disturbance in Pitta or Kapha dosha. By changing her diet and adopting various other health routines that help balance these two doshas, Amy was able to make remarkable progress in a short time. In the first three months after beginning the treatments offered by Maharishi Vedic Medicine, she had only one mild episode of urinary tract infection, which lasted less than forty-eight hours. Moreover, her backache completely disappeared, and she started having more energy. In her own words, she felt wonderful. After more than two years, Amy remains quite healthy and continues to use Maharishi Vedic Medicine for prevention.

Amy's experience illustrates something important. Although she sought treatment for her recurring infections, once the doshic imbalances underlying that condition started to clear up, her other symptoms disappeared as well. Physicians practicing Maharishi Vedic Medicine time and again have this experience—unrelated surface symptoms disappear when their primary cause is removed.

Imbalanced Doshas: The First Step Toward Illness

Everything you do affects your body and the doshas that govern your body's functions. The food you eat, your waking and sleeping habits, all elements of your behavior affect the doshas. Maharishi Vedic Medicine uses the principle of similarities and opposites to explain this process. According to this principle, influences that have qualities similar to those of a specific dosha increase that dosha, while influences that have opposite qualities bring about its decrease.[15]

Numerous disorders and diseases result from long-term lifestyle habits that aggravate a particular dosha continuously over time. For example Vata dosha is associated with movement and with quick, dry, and light qualities. If you eat mainly foods that are dry and light—like lots of crackers or granola—these foods will increase Vata in the body. If you eat foods that are oily, heavy, and dense, that is, opposite in quality to Vata, Vata will decrease.*

Three States of the Doshas [16]

Balanced (sama)	This state represents the normal functioning of the doshas.
Increase, aggravation (vriddhi)	At this stage, different physiological or mental symptoms manifest, depending on the amount of aggravation.
Decrease (kshina)	Decrease of normal functioning of the doshas.

---

*On the other hand, eating or doing almost anything in excess can disturb Vata.

Factors that Aggravate the Doshas

Vata	*Pitta*	*Kapha*
Foods		
•Rough, dry, light, astringent, bitter, and pungent foods	•Hot, sharp, sour, acidic, salty, and pungent foods	• Heavy, oily, cold, sweet, sour, salty, sticky foods
•Fasting, eating too little, losing too much weight	•Skipping meals	•Eating too much food
Behavior		
•Mental or physical exertion (working long hours, exercising too much, traveling, speaking, straining, getting fatigued)	•Bone fractures, injuries	•Alcohol and cigarettes
	•Overexertion (speaking, working, or thinking too much)	•Resting and sleeping too much, especially during the daytime and after meals
•Suppressing natural urges (e.g., to urinate, sneeze, or have bowel movements)	•Excessive exposure to heat or sunshine	• Lack of exercise
•Not getting enough sleep	•Fasting	
•Keeping an irregular routine (eating at different times every day, going to bed at different times)		
Emotions		
•Fear, grief, worry anxiety, agitation, anger	•Anger, hatred, jealously, passion	•Possessiveness, greed
Weather		
•Dry, cold, windy, and changeable weather	•Hot weather	•Cold, wet weather

Eating a meal of spicy, sharp, and acidic foods would increase the spicy, sharp, acidic, fiery qualities of Pitta, while eating cooling foods such as milk and ghee would decrease them.

In other words, to understand how the doshas get imbalanced and rebalanced, simply remember that like increases like, while opposites tend to neutralize or balance each other. For this reason, it's not only the quality of the foods you eat that influences the doshas, but also the quality of your activity. A person working in a fast-food restaurant, for example, must work very quickly and efficiently. Because Vata is associated both with movements and quick, sudden changes, such activity would surely increase Vata dosha over time. Conversely, getting a good night's sleep would decrease Vata.

If you lose touch with the body's underlying intelligence, you lose your natural sensitivity to your body and its needs. As a consequence, you make mistakes in diet or daily routine, eating foods or engaging in work that disturbs the natural, constitutional balance of the doshas. Then, doshic imbalances start to creep in. At first, this does not necessarily manifest as disease. In the first stages of imbalance, you might simply feel the difference as a lack of your well-being. If Vata dosha is balanced, for example, you'll feel creative and quick-thinking. However, if the innate equilibrium of Vata is lost, these positive qualities get distorted. You worry or feel anxious, lose too much weight or have trouble sleeping at night.

Each dosha is associated with an area of the body called its "seat." A doshic imbalance will initially show up in this area, since it is where that dosha is centered. The main seat of Vata is the large intestine. Pitta is found in the small intestine. Kapha is found in the stomach. These three primary seats, located in the gastrointestinal tract, are known as the *koshtha*. As long as the doshas stay in the koshtha they remain relatively harmless, because the excess energy of any one dosha can easily flow out of the body through the elimination system.

The disease process starts if the imbalanced dosha spreads to another part of the body and begins to accumulate there. This happens when the natural flow of the body's inherent intelligence becomes disrupted because of unhealthy diet, daily routine, unhealthy behaviors, excessive exercise, and so on. The mental pressure resulting from deadlines, hectic work habits, or the hyperactive mental activity associated with imbalanced Vata can also trigger this process.[17] In addition, unhealthy digestion plays a key role in the spread of the doshas outside their normal domains. This will be the focus of the next chapter.

Because Vata dosha is associated with movement, it plays a major role in the flow of the doshas through the mind-body. It is the least stable of the three doshas and therefore quick to go out of balance. When Vata becomes imbalanced, the pressure of excess Vata sooner or later will cause the other doshas to leave the koshtha and localize elsewhere in the body. This is why Vata dosha has the dubious distinction of being known as the king dosha—it moves the other two.

Each dosha has several subdivisions or subdoshas, as described in Chapter 3, and a disease often involves one or several of these. Rheumatoid arthritis, for example, is linked to an imbalance in no less than five subdoshas: Vyana Vata, which is involved in circulation; Shleshaka Kapha, which is responsible for the lubrication of joints; Kledaka Kapha, which is associated with the functioning of the stomach; Pachaka Pitta, which is seated in the small intestine; and Samana Vata, which helps stimulate the digestive fluids.

Doshic imbalance can progress into disease in two ways, gradually or suddenly.

Gradual

In this scenario, disease develops through the gradual accumulation of excess doshas over time. If you eat a large quantity of

---

Diseases Associated with Imbalance in the Subdoshas
Subdoshas of Vata

Prana	Respiratory disorders, cognitive problems, neurological disorders
Udana	Diseases of the nose, throat, speech, ears
Samana	Anorexia; irregular, weak digestion
Apana	Constipation, diarrhea, menstrual problems, sexual dysfunction
Vyana	Circulatory and heart disease; many other diseases

Subdoshas of Pitta

Pachaka	Imbalance in digestion; anemia, jaundice
Ranjaka	Anemia and other blood disorders
Sadhaka	Decreased decisiveness, intelligence, and memory; affective psychiatric disorders (depression, etc.)
Alochaka	Visual problems
Bhrajaka	Skin diseases

Subdoshas of Kapha

Kledaka	Dull digestion; effect on all other Kaphas
Avalambaka	Back pain, heart problems
Bodhaka	Disruption of taste
Tarpaka	Sinus problems, nasal congestion, cough coming from upper respiratory tract, problems with senses
Shleshaka	Joint problems

---

heavy, oily foods for several days, for example, it can produce a mild increase in Kapha in the stomach. If you adjust your diet, your body most likely will be able to normalize the resulting Kapha increase by itself. However, if you continue to eat these Kapha-aggravating foods, the imbalance not only will remain, but also will intensify over time. Eventually, if you don't change your eating habits somewhere along the way, the aggravation of Kapha will result in manifest signs of disease. The excess doshas will move from their seats in the digestive tract to any weak tissues in the body. If the joints are weak, the excess doshas could move there and create stiff joints or arthritis. If the lungs are weak, the doshas might move there, creating breathing disturbances or other problems.

Sudden

A sudden shock to your emotions, such as news of the death of a loved one or a sudden loss in business, can cause an abrupt increase and aggravation of Vata dosha. This can rapidly spread to other areas and create faintness, mental instability, and depression. The progression of disease follows the same sequence, but happens so suddenly that the different stages are not easily detectable.

In most cases, diseases result from the *gradual* accumulation of doshic imbalances in the body. The excess doshas can circulate in the body tissues for quite a while before developing into a disease. If the imbalance is mild and the natural strength of the body is strong, then the inherent self-regulating intelligence of the body can usually correct the imbalance and halt the progression of disease. If the imbalance is moderate or severe, however, therapeutic measures need to be applied to prevent it from causing disruption to the body's tissues.

Once the vitiated doshas spread to the tissues, you start experiencing the first physical signs of the disturbance. As you'll recall from Chapter 3, in Maharishi Vedic Medicine the body tissues are referred to as the dhatus, and disease can be understood entirely in terms of their condition. As the *Charaka Samhita* states, "Any disturbance in the equilibrium of the dhatus is known as disease, and on the other hand, the state of their equilibrium is health."[18]

The healthy functioning of the body's tissues depends on the activity of the doshas. The balanced functioning of the doshas ensures the proper maintenance of the dhatus and the integrity of their activity. However, when the doshas go out of balance, the imbalance often spreads to the dhatus, resulting in dysfunction and disease. Arthritis, for example, is characterized by a swelling of the joints and is associated with malfunctioning in the muscle and bone tissue. Anemia is characterized by a dysfunction in the blood. In Maharishi Vedic Medicine the blood is considered a body tissue.

The combination of imbalanced doshas and abnormal dhatus is one of the most decisive developments in the gradual break-down of the body's natural equilibrium. Once the disease process reaches this level, it is much harder to reverse. This explains why Maharishi Vedic Medicine places such great emphasis on eliminating imbalances in the mind-body long before they show up as disturbances on the level of the tissues. The disease process also involves disturbance of a number of other body functions, which will be considered in the following two chapters.

CHAPTER 7

The Drama of Agni, Ama and Ojas

"The nourishment of the dhatus, ojas, strength, complexion, etc., by food depends on *agni*; because *rasa* etc. (the seven dhatus) cannot be produced from undigested food." —*Charaka Samhita*[19]

When Jane first sought treatment at the Maharishi Vedic Medical Center, she had severe constipation and was unable to move her bowels more than once or twice a week. For several years, she had suffered from dizziness and depression, as well as gas and bloating after eating. The symptoms had spread to pain in her knees, hip joints and lower back. She was also having extreme hot flashes from menopause and fluid retention in her legs and breasts. The hot flashes prevented her from sleeping peacefully, and her nights were disturbed and agitated. As if all this wasn't enough, she was also experiencing constant headaches and congested nose and sinuses. She had gone from physician to physician in a desperate search for help, but the treatments her doctors had prescribed had provided little relief.

Considering the range and severity of her ailments, Jane at first stared in disbelief at me when, instead of prescribing yet another drug, I recommended some simple lifestyle changes to improve her condition. I put her on a diet that would help balance her doshas and that emphasized foods that were easy for her to digest, and I gave her some herbal food supplements to stimulate digestion and elimination. I also gave her some mind-body exercises to increase physical relaxation and harmony, and recommended that she start the Transcendental Meditation technique to reduce mental stress. After just a few weeks, her condition dramatically improved. Jane reported a noticeable increase in her energy level, and the gas and bloating disappeared. Over the next three to four months, her constipation disappeared and she started having a daily bowel movement. Once her digestive problems started to clear up, the other ailments diminished. Her sleep became normal, her headaches subsided, her fluid retention was minimal, and her sinus problem completely disappeared. In one year's time, Jane recovered her health and sense of well-being.

Jane's main problem was poor digestion. Of course, the bloating, gas, and constipation she experienced were clear signs of a digestive disorder. But the joint pain, headaches, sinus congestion, and loss of appetite were also related to her digestive difficulties. These conditions have their source in or are aggravated by improperly digested food. Therefore, it is a common experience that once digestive problems are addressed, a whole gamut of symptoms starts to disappear.

Digestion is the central player in gaining or maintaining perfect health. According to Maharishi Vedic Medicine, the balance or imbalance of the doshas is linked to the relative strength or weakness of the digestive fire. Fire is one of Nature's five basic elements. In the human body, fire or heat takes the form of the digestive liquids, known as agni. The heat of agni corresponds to the sun. Agni has the qualities of heat and transformation, like a flame of fire, or the sun itself.

On a day-to-day basis, the processes of eating, metabolizing, and eliminating constitute the most important means to upholding the health and vitality of the body. Diet is one of the three pillars of life (along with proper sleep and meditation) and one of the most important therapeutic modalities. The right foods eaten at the right time in the right amounts provide a powerful tool for normalizing the doshas and restoring health. Virtually any illness can be treated and prevented by balancing the digestive fire.

Maharishi Vedic Medicine is unique in its focus on digestive health. If you went to a medical doctor and told him that you wanted to improve your digestion, he would probably ask you if you were having pain in your stomach. If so, he would assume you had an ulcer, irritable bowel syndrome, or colon cancer. If you had none of these diseases, he'd probably tell you your digestion was just fine, or he might suggest that your problems were psychological in origin. Western medicine focuses almost exclusively on overt symptoms of disorders. Maharishi Vedic Medicine aims at addressing disorders long before they reach such a late stage in the disease process. Maharishi Vedic Medicine traces many disorders to unhealthy digestion. The strength of your agni, or digestive fire affects your overall mental and physical health. The *Charaka Samhita* states, "Strength, health, longevity and vital breath are dependent upon the power of digestion (agni)."[20]

The Ayurvedic texts provide important insights into the subtle steps through which the digestive process unfolds. The process of eating is actually one of ingesting orderliness from the environment—you take in concentrated packets of intelligence to feed or support the body's intelligence. It's important to understand the details of this digestive process so that you can work with it rather than against it.

The Thirteen Agnis and Their Functions

One of the main branches of Ayurvedic treatment is called *kayachikitsa*, or "therapy of fire." *Kaya* means "fire" and *chikitsa* "therapy of." Kayachikitsa is all about sustaining and balancing the digestive fire, agni. Fire is one of the five elements that make up not only your body but the "body" of the universe as well. Agni has the qualities of heat and transformation, just like the flame of a fire. Agni's transformational capacity facilitates all growth processes in living systems. For example, in the human body, agni can appear in the form of digestive secretions, which change food into something the body can assimilate and use.

There are thirteen different qualities of agni, each of which plays a certain role in transforming food into the body's tissues. The main location of agni is in the digestive juices in the large and small intestines and the stomach. These secretions are called *jatharagni*, and they are responsible for converting the food you eat into the nutrient plasma that circulates throughout the body and nourishes all the cells and tissues.

Jatharagni is made up of five *bhutagnis*. They represent each of the five elements of Nature (earth, water, fire, air, space) and help to digest food made up of the corresponding element. Even though all five elements form jatharagni, it is mainly fire. Though a liquid, it is not moist. Rather it is like a cooking fire, and is responsible for cooking or digesting the food.

Seven Dhatu Agnis

In addition to these six agnis (jatharagni and the five bhutagnis), each of the seven body tissues, or dhatus, has an associated agni. These agnis help transform one tissue into the other in the sequential process of digestion. Each *dhatu agni* is highly specific in its function as it converts its "assigned" dhatu into the next one in the cycle.

The thirteen agnis work in an orderly progression to digest the food you eat. When you eat a carrot, jatharagni "cooks" or transforms the food into two substances. One could be called the nutritional essence itself (*prasad*), that will be digested or metabolized into progressively more refined substances as it travels into finer and finer levels of the physiology. The other substance (*kitt*) is basically waste matter, which will continue moving along through the digestive tract. Despite their general differences, prasad and kitt will still yield both nutritive matter and waste matter as they undergo further steps of digestion, transformation, and metabolism. The next step is for the prasad to be digested by the five bhutagnis and converted into rasa dhatu, the first tissue of the body, as well as into the inevitable waste products, or malas, that result from every digestive transformation. The seven dhatu agnis continue the conversion process, working in a fixed sequence with their associated tissues, to complete digestion.

Once you understand the critical role agni plays in nourishing each dhatu, you can see why maintaining the digestive fire is essential for health. For example, a disturbance in meda agni—which is located in the dhatu concerned with body fat—may cause you to gain too much weight. A disturbance in rakta agni could cause a blood disorder.

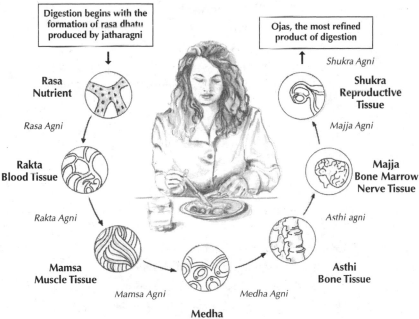

Digestion begins with the formation of rasa dhatu produced by jatharagni

Ojas, the most refined product of digestion

Shukra Agni

Rasa
Nutrient

Shukra
Reproductive
Tissue

Rasa Agni

Majja Agni

Rakta
Blood Tissue

Majja
Bone Marrow
Nerve Tissue

Rakta Agni

Asthi agni

Mamsa
Muscle Tissue

Asthi
Bone Tissue

Mamsa Agni

Medha Agni

Medha
Fat Tissue

How Imbalanced Jatharagni Leads to Disease

The strength of the dhatu agnis depends on the strength of jatharagni. If jatharagni is strong and in balance, then the dhatu agnis will be strong and in balance. A balanced jatharagni produces a clear, thin, odorless, unctuous nutrient fluid, called *rasa dhatu*. Rasa dhatu is the first product of digested food. When it is properly digested, it nourishes all the other dhatus, and is capable of entering the smallest pores of the body to provide nutrition to the tiniest cell. Rasa dhatu, the nutrient material, nourishes

---

Signs of Strong Agni

Clear complexion	Clarity of mind	Good voice
Energy	Genius	Happiness
Satisfaction	Nourishment	Strength
Strong intellect	Long life span	Health
Enthusiasm	Luster	

Signs of Weak Agni

Dullness	Bloating	Gas
Heartburn	Lack of energy	Heaviness
Giddiness	Dizziness	Light-headedness
Pain	Bad taste in mouth	Bad breath

Factors that Derange Agni

Fasting

Overeating

Irregular eating

Eating before previous meal is digested

Eating during indigestion

Eating unwholesome food

Suppression of natural urges

Faulty administration of eliminative procedures

Faulty adaptation to place, climate, season

Negative emotions, such as anger, worry, sorrow, fear

---

and builds all the body tissues. It circulates throughout the body, supplying nutrients to each tissue as it is sequentially converted into the other tissues.

When jatharagni is weak or out of balance, it does not break down the food properly, and unhealthy or unusable nutrient materials are created. For example, weak or dull agni produces undigested or inadequately digested food. On the other hand, if agni is too strong, it burns or chars the food, as if you burned the food on your stove. And erratic agni produces a mixture of digested and undigested food.

Ama: The Precursor of Disease

Each of these three abnormal digestive p atterns (weak, too strong, erratic) creates *ama*, the remains of undigested food. Ama is a sticky, bad-smelling, toxic substance. Ama is different from the malas, the normal waste produced by healthy digestion.

When digestion is weak, ama gets mixed in the rasa dhatu, the nutrient fluid, and circulates throughout the body. When agni is imbalanced, large amounts of ama are produced, resulting in a thick, cloudy, sticky, foul-smelling nutrient fluid that cannot pass through minute pores because it is full of heavy impurities. As you can imagine, this polluted nutrient fluid cannot nourish the dhatus properly. It cannot reach the tissue cells, and instead accumulates outside them and distorts the dhatus with swelling.

Ama also clogs the body's channels—the arteries, veins and lymphatic system—as well as the channels of the dhatus and pores. By obstructing these vital pipelines for communication and nourishment, ama inhibits physiological functioning. Ama can also form a coating on the walls of the body's channels, stopping fluids from moving freely. Finally, it can damage or cut off the cell's connection with its source in Nature's intelligence. This destructive influence of ama can cause many diseases, from arteriosclerosis to arthritis to Alzheimer's.

How Ama Mixes with the Doshas and Creates Disease

As ama gets mixed with the nutrient fluids and travels through-out the body, it generates many symptoms. As it blocks the physi-ological passages and cell pores, the individual experiences a loss of strength and feels heavy. Signs of increased ama include dimin-ished activity of Vata dosha, lethargy, indigestion, expectoration of phlegm, accumulation of waste materials in the body, loss of taste and appetite, and exhaustion.

The three doshas are present in the nutrient fluid (rasa dhatu). Consequently, they get mixed with ama and become dis-torted by its impurities. These abnormal doshas enter into the body tissues and waste products, giving rise to many illnesses. Dis-ease symptoms take on the qualities of the doshas. For example, Vata dosha combined with ama creates constipation, poor diges-tive activity, intestinal gurgling, pain, and swelling. Pitta dosha mixed with ama produces a sour taste, burning sensations in the throat and heart, thirst, and sour, heavy elimination. Kapha and ama produce a buildup of thready, foul-smelling, thick mucous in the throat, and loss of hunger.

How Ama Affects the Seven Dhatu Agnis

The seven dhatu agnis are responsible for digestion and the separation of nutrient and waste material. These agnis, when strong, lead to normal development and vitality in the dhatus. Therefore, good health depends on the health of the dhatu agnis.

You'll remember that the strength of the dhatu agnis depends mainly on the strength and balance of jatharagni. A weak jathar-agni causes weak dhatu agnis, which results in the production and accumulation of ama in the tissues. The dhatus then swell with impurities. A different problem is caused when a sharp, strong jatharagni and dhatu agnis cause the nutrients to be di-gested too quickly. The dhatu agnis then start digesting the tis-sues, leading to depletion, destruction, or loss of the tissues. Ama is also generated in the tissues by the combination of imbalanced doshas and dhatus. All these accumulations of ama in the tissues generate chronic diseases.

Ojas: The Harbinger of Health

When digestion is strong, the body produces an abundance of a substance called *ojas*. This vital material results from healthy diet, digestion, behavior, and mental and emotional states. People with a lot of ojas often have a bright, luminous complexion—the proverbial glow of health.

Ama and ojas have opposite effects on the body. Ama obstructs the flow of intelligence in the body, whereas ojas aids it. Ojas is considered to be the finest material form of consciousness. It exists at the fine junction point where the totally abstract, unmanifest field of consciousness first expresses itself as matter. Ojas pervades the body, residing in the gaps between the body tissues. When ojas is lively in your physiology, it affects all aspects of the mind-body, creating enthusiasm, knowledge, and understanding; fullness of feeling on the level of the mind; nourishment; and complete health on the level of the physiology. Insufficient ojas results in emaciation, laziness, impotency, ignorance, and confusion.

Ojas is similar to balanced Kapha in quality. It is heavy, cold, soft, smooth, thick, sweet, stable, clear, sticky, and unctuous. Ojas is found in two forms. One kind of ojas is present in each of the dhatus and in the organs composed of the dhatus. It constitutes the essence of the dhatus. It is responsible for strength, stability, good muscular development, the capacity for physical work, and efficient working of the senses and the mind. It also bestows good voice and complexion. The other kind of ojas is present in the heart, in the form of eight drops. Here, it is slightly red or yellow in color. If lost or damaged, it leads to loss of life itself.

Ojas and Immunity

Ojas is intimately linked with the strength or immunity of the body, called *bala*. Physiological vitality is directly correlated with the quantity of ojas present. Sufficient ojas in the body tissues keeps the doshas from distorting the dhatus, and it prevents the union of abnormal doshas and dhatus. It creates resistance to any influence that might bring about dysfunction in the dhatus. If ojas decreases in quantity or quality, the dhatus become more vulnerable to imbalanced doshas and other factors that produce disease. Once imbalanced, the dhatus increase or decrease resulting in many types of illness.

When ojas is available in normal quantities, it prevents imbalance in the dhatus, doshas and agnis, which means it helps prevent the onset of disease within the body. Ojas also helps the body withstand disease from the outside. That is why the entire purpose of Maharishi Vedic Medicine is to maintain a physiological state in which ojas is constantly generated and maintained.

Fluctuations in Ojas

Ojas is present in differing amounts, depending on the individual's doshic constitution, the seasons of the year, and the time of life. For all people, though, the more ojas present in the body, the healthier they will be.

What causes ojas to increase? While ama is the product of undigested food, ojas is the most refined product of digestion. The food you eat gets sequentially transformed by the dhatus. The dhatus, you'll remember, are formed by the seven dhatu agnis. Ojas is created as a result of each dhatu formation, and is also the end-product of *shukra* tissue. (Shukra is the final product of the chain of digestion.) Since ojas is the product of digestion, the foods you eat figure heavily in its generation. Some foods are especially nourishing, such as milk, butter, and *ghee* (clarified butter).

These foods create ojas almost immediately. If the food you eat is old, left over, full of chemicals, difficult to digest, or unsuitable for your doshas, it will not yield much ojas.

How Ojas Gets Destroyed

When ojas decreases, the body becomes weak, disease can develop, and the life span is shortened. If ojas is sufficiently diminished, this can lead to death. In general, a moderate lifestyle and eating habits promote ojas, while eating the wrong kinds of foods and following an unhealthy routine destroy it. The actions that particularly destroy ojas include injury; harm to the body; weight loss; excessive anger, grief, thinking, worry, anxiety, physical activity, and hunger; staying awake at night; the consumption of dry foods and alcohol; too little food or the absence of food; taking in poisons, such as tobacco, prescribed or nonprescribed drugs, or even excessive amounts of coffee or tea; and too much elimination of Kapha dosha, blood, semen, or waste products.

Good Health and Happiness

In this chapter, you have seen that agni and ama are the main players in the daily drama of digestion. Agni, the digestive fire, is the luminous hero of the story. When agni is burning brightly and steadily, then digestion is normal. When agni is weak for any reason, then ama starts to accumulate in the digestive tract. Ama's qualities are opposite to those of the fiery agni. Ama is undigested food. Cold, sticky, and heavy, a toxic waste-product of digestion, ama collects in the tissues and creates trouble wherever it spreads.

If your digestion is irregular or interrupted in some way, ama is created instead of the nutrients that nourish the body's tissues and sustain life. These toxic impurities form in the stomach, dhatus, and cells. Ama can travel to any part of the body, clogging or deforming channels such as the arteries and creating weakness wherever it goes. It tends to build up, causing further disruption to the affected channels. Eventually activity in the body's passages changes from orderly to disorderly to disconnected from Nature's intelligence. The organ that is fed by those channels (for example, in the case of arteries, the heart) gets destroyed.

When the body is coherent—when the doshas, dhatus, agnis, and ojas are balanced—bliss is the result. Ojas could be said to be the material form of bliss. When ojas is at an optimal level in the body, you feel happy and contented and you are free of illness. Like Jane—who found that improved digestion was the key to correcting a myriad of problems, from hot flashes to insomnia to backache—you may find that balancing your digestion can liberate you from a wide range of disorders.

CHAPTER 8

The Srotas: Your Physiological Transportation System

> "Food and regimen that aggravate the doshas are
> contrary to the well-being of the dhatus and vitiate the
> channels (*srotas*)."
> —*Charaka Samhita*[21]

One of the fascinating facts about the human body is that it is not a solid mass. It is composed of innumerable tissue cells, which are interconnected by thousands of channels of circulation, communication and nourishment. You can also think of these channels as gateways or passages that connect the tissue cells. The body is made up mostly of these empty spaces.

These channels, called *srotas*, can either be quite large or so small that they are virtually invisible. The srotas are defined as any space inside the body—channels, veins, arteries, lymph passages, ducts, residences, sites, containers and abodes. Some srotas are large and noticeable. These include the two nostrils, the tear ducts in the eyes, the two ears, the mouth, the urethra, and the colon. These nine large passageways are called external srotas, because they have a visible opening to the outside of the body. Their specific purposes are to move materials in and out of the body.

Most srotas are so minute that they can't be seen at all. They are part of the body's tissue, and are composed of the same elements as the tissue itself. The tissue cells are constantly rebuilding themselves, importing nutrient fluid and exporting wastes. Each tissue cell is composed of thousands of tiny srotas, and these channels carry the nutrient fluids and the nutrients undergoing transformation to each cell. They also carry waste products away from the cells.

Srotas can be visible or invisible to the naked eye, round, circular, thick or thin, long, or similar to the network of ribs in a leaf. They are usually the same color as the dhatu in which they are found, only paler, and they are named after that dhatu. Thus the muscle tissue (*mamsa dhatu*) contains channels called *mamsavaha srota*; the srotas in bone tissue (*asthid hatu*) are called *asthivaha srota*, and so on.

How the Srotas Work

The srotas have amazingly precise tasks. They will not allow just any fluid to pass through them. Only the specific nutrient that they are designed to carry can move through. For example, the srotas in the muscle tissue will only allow nutrient materials necessary to form muscle tissue to flow through them. The srotas are dhatu-specific, and the work of one srota cannot be done by another.

Once nutrients reach the cells via the srotas, they are metabolized or digested by the dhatu agni, the distinct form of digestive fluid that transforms nutrient material into a particular tissue. The dhatu agni produces three materials: (1) nutrition for the dhatu, which stays in the cell to nourish it and form new tissue; (2) nutrition for the next dhatu, which moves out of the cell and is circulated to the next tissue to use via the rasa dhatu; and (3) waste products, which are also circulated through the rasa dhatu. As materials move in and out of tissue cells via the srotas, they facilitate digestion of nutrient fluid, dhatu growth and development, formation of the next dhatu in the sequence of transformation, and elimination of waste. Each of these functions is part of tissue metabolism, and the srotas are the channels that allow the necessary exchanges to take place. All the srotas also serve as

The Types of Srotas[22]

Intake Srotas

1. Channels that transport breath, or prana: respiratory system (pranavaha srotas)
2. Channels that transport food: digestive system (annavaha srotas)
3. Channels that transport water and control water metabolism: digestive system (ambuvaha srotas)

Dhatu Srotas

4. Channels that transport plasma to blood and tissue: lymphatic and circulatory systems (rasavaha srotas)
5. Channels that transport blood and hemoglobin: circulatory system (raktavaha srotas)
6. Channels that nourish the muscle tissues: muscular system (mamsavaha srotas)
7. Channels that nourish the fat tissues: adipose system (medavaha srotas)
8. Channels that supply the bones: skeletal system (asthivaha srotas)
9. Channels that supply the bone marrow, nerve and brain tissue: nervous system (majjavaha srotas)
10. Channels that nourish and govern the reproductive tissue (in males this specifically includes semen): reproductive system (shukravaha srotas)

Waste Removal Srotas

11. Channels that carry urine: urinary system (mutravaha srotas)
12. Channels that carry feces, excrement: excretory system (purishavaha srotas)
13. Channels that carry sweat: sebaceous system (svedavaha srotas)

Srotas for the Female System

14. Channels that carry menstrual blood: female reproductive system (artavavaha srotas)
15. Channels that carry milk during lactation: female hormonal system

channels for the movement of the doshas throughout the body.

The body contains thirteen different types of srotas, located in the respiratory, lymphatic, and digestive systems, as well as in the dhatus and eliminative organs. Women have two additional srota networks involved in lactation and menstruation.

How the Srotas Become Obstructed

Improper food and daily routines are the main causes of distortion in the activity of the srotas. Poor diet and routine aggravate the doshas and disrupt the well-being of the dhatus. Overeating, eating before the previous meal is digested, eating unwholesome and incompatible foods, sleeping after meals, engaging in too much or too little exercise, weak agni, excessive heat or shock, and engaging in excessive worry are all influences that distort or disrupt the srotas.[23]

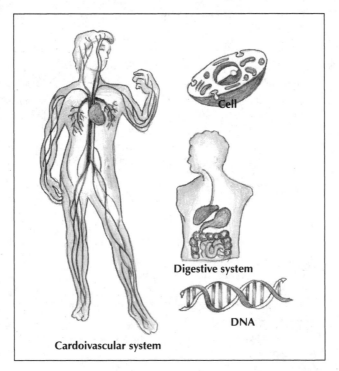

Cell

Digestive system

DNA

Cardoivascular system

The doshas and dhatus are considered normal if they exist in the proper quantity and maintain their proper qualities and functions. The health of tissue cells, srotas, and the organs that make up the thirteen srota systems is also judged in terms of proper quantity, quality and function. Four types of imbalances can disrupt the srotas and each can lead to different types of diseases.

Excessive flow

This is characterized by increased activity of the organs of the system. In the respiratory system, it could cause faster breathing; in the circulatory system, faster heartbeat. Diarrhea, sweating, and increased frequency of urination are other examples of this type of imbalance.

Obstructed flow

The organs slow down due to obstruction of the srotas caused by ama. As a result, the organs swell, shrink, or change shape. Initially, obstruction of the srotas could make an organ work faster or slower. Eventually, it causes the breakdown of the organ. Arteriosclerosis, commonly known as hardening of the arteries, is an example of blockage in the channels leading to the heart. The heart slows down, becomes enlarged, and functions at a handicap. If the lung's air passages become clogged, breathing slows down. Constipation, congested sinuses, or blocked urination provide other examples. This is the most common type of imbalanced srota, and it occurs when disease becomes localized in one place and can be identified. Disease means that a srota is blocked.

Reversed or diverted flow

In a healthy person, the fluids moving in and out of the tissue cells have a fixed path. However, if ama clogs the srota, fluids can start to move up when they're supposed to move down, or can get diverted to another srota. Vomiting, a sour taste in the mouth after burping (hyperacidity), and jaundice (yellow bile enters the blood stream) are all examples of reversed or diverted flow in the srotas.

Structural changes

This kind of abnormality causes the tissue cells to increase their size and shape. Benign and malignant tumors, growths, moles, warts, and nodules can develop in the srotas or organs.

Of these four abnormalities, the majority of diseases result from obstruction, and ama is its major cause. Ama, the sticky, unusable waste product of undigested food, is produced by weak digestive fire (agni) or by imbalances in the seven tissues (dhatu agnis) when they metabolize nutrient material. Once ama is created, it mixes with the nutrient materials and circulates all over the body, spreading to dhatus and tissue cells through the srotas.

When nutrient material (rasa) is combined with ama, it takes on a different quality. It becomes thick and heavy, and it jams the srotas. You could think of it like dirty oil, which gums up your car engine and clogs the hoses and tubes. When ama chokes the srotas, they swell and the dhatus get bigger. When ama accumulates, it blocks proper nutrition to the cells, and the srotas and dhatus can no longer function properly. Wherever ama gathers, it is often accompanied by pain. Pain is a sign of the buildup of ama in the tissues, pores and srotas.

One of the most destructive effects of distorted srota activity is the inhibition of the flow of ojas in the body. Ojas is a prime contributor to immunity. It prevents disease, nourishes the dhatus and creates bliss in the mind and body. Maharishi Vedic Medicine focuses on clearing the srotas of toxins and strengthening digestion, because these two measures keep ojas flowing and avert illness.

CHAPTER 9

The Six Stages of Disease

"The entire body is in fact the abode of all the three doshas, viz., Vata, Pitta and Kapha, and as such these doshas bring about good and bad results according as they are in normal and abnormal states respectively. When in a normal state they bring about good results like growth, strength, complexion, happiness, etc. When in an abnormal state, they cause various types of diseases.... Diseases caused by Vata are of eighty types, those by Pitta of forty types and those by Kapha of twenty types."
—*Charaka Samhita*[24]

Joan's physician explained that her chronic fatigue was due to overwork. Each night she'd tumble into bed exhausted, with every part of her body aching, only to find that she couldn't sleep. Hiatal hernia and gastroesophageal reflux disease, for which she took prescribed medicine, created painful burning in her esophagus at night, contributing to her insomnia. She started developing headaches and depression for the first time, and remembers trying to explain this to her physician: "I'm embarrassed to tell you this. It's kind of vague but very real, too." She knew something was severely out of balance, but her physician could find no cause, so she decided to wait until her retirement, when the extra rest would surely cure her.

She became alarmed when, a few months after retirement, she still couldn't shake the symptoms. After seeking help at a Maharishi Vedic Medical Center, Joan started practicing the Transcendental Meditation technique regularly, adjusted her diet to balance the doshas, and started taking Maharishi Ayur-Veda herbs for the hiatal hernia. Just one year later, Joan is sleeping at night and no longer has gastrointestinal problems. Nor does she need medication for them. She is free of headaches and has the energy she used to enjoy. "I don't know how to say it, but everything is better and more beautiful," she said. "I get up in the morning and I have the energy to take care of my garden and everything around me. The change has been dramatic."

So many times, a patient comes to a doctor and says, "I just don't feel right." Yet, unless there is a definable, organic cause for the problem, modern medical tests usually cannot diagnose it. In Joan's case, for example, she thinks her gastrointestinal problem started five years before it was diagnosed properly. "I had sonograms and tests for gall bladder, but that wasn't the problem. Finally, when the symptoms got to be so classic, my physician recommended x-rays and identified the problem."

However, it is at the stage when you "just don't feel right" that disease can be prevented and most easily cured. It is well documented that chronic disease takes many months and even years to develop. Diseases start as a small imbalance, but if they remain unchecked they move step-by-step into a full-blown illness, such as heart disease, hypertension or chronic fatigue.

Fortunately, Maharishi Vedic Medicine is able to diagnose imbalances long before they manifest as significant symptoms. In fact, by the time the body shows clear signs of illness, the disorder is in its final stages, not the beginning. This chapter looks at how a disease can start as an uncomfortable feeling and progress to obvious, fully developed symptoms.

Six Stages in the Progression of an Imbalance

So far you have learned that pragya-aparadh, the mistake of the intellect, is the source of most diseases. You've also seen how eating the wrong foods and following an unhealthy routine can

---

The Pathophysiology of Disease

Doshas	+	**Agni**	+	**Srotas**
increased,		weak, dull, or		widened, obstructed
decreased,		excessive–		nodular, or reversed
or vitiated		creates ama		flow

---

cause imbalances in the three doshas, the three basic physiological operators. Distorted doshic activity produces distortion in the tissues. Weak digestion also contributes to disease by generating toxins, called ama, which circulate throughout the body. The spread of ama impairs immunity (associated with ojas), blocks the body's channels of transportation and communication (srotas), and prevents the tissue cells (dhatus) from receiving proper nourishment.

Now it's important to understand how these different contributors to illness work together. In analyzing disease, Maharishi Vedic Medicine identifies six distinct stages: accumulation, aggravation, dissemination, localization, manifestation, and disruption.

Stage 1 Accumulation: The doshas accumulate in their own sites.

Stage 2 Aggravation: The doshas become imbalanced or vitiated, which creates a spur to move out of their normal sites.

Stage 3 Dissemination: The imbalanced doshas migrate to other parts of the body.

Stage 4 Localization: The doshas combine with ama in a particular organ or tissue and concentrate there.

Stage 5 Manifestation: The disease manifests as specific signs and symptoms.

Stage 6 Disruption: The disease progresses from acute to chronic, or else moves into complications.

Patients generally don't know what is happening in stages one to four. When they get to stages five and six, they usually feel motivated to go to a doctor. Unfortunately, by then it is almost too late, because once clear symptoms arise, the disease can be difficult to cure or control. Maharishi Vedic Medicine tries to handle the situation in stages one to three, before the disorder displays obvious symptoms. In stages one or two, the doshas remain in their natural locations, and structural changes in the tissues—which can be irreversible—have not yet occurred.

Stage One: Accumulation

The doshas are not stable in quantity, quality or function. They are affected by the foods you eat and by your environment, behavior, thoughts, emotions, and waking and sleeping routines. One inevitable cause of doshic imbalance is the yearly cycle of seasons. In the heat of summer, fiery Pitta starts to accumulate and can cause skin rashes, anger or other Pitta-related problems. In winter, cold, dry Vata increases, causing colds, anxiety or arthritis. In spring, the influence of cool, wet, heavy Kapha becomes stronger, and can lead to coughs, weight gain and flu.

As part of the yearly cycle, the doshas tend to aggregate over two to four months. You don't have to suffer from these effects, though, as Maharishi Vedic Medicine prescribes special dietary guidelines and behaviors to counteract doshic imbalances during each season. In the winter, for example, if you eat foods that are opposite in quality to Vata, you can keep it from increasing. You can also take advantage of a purification procedure, called Maharishi Rejuvenation therapy. This includes steam baths, heat treatments and intestinal cleansers to sweep away impurities at the end of every season. That way, you can prevent an unhealthy doshic buildup.

Doshas also accumulate from eating foods or engaging in activities that are not suitable for your nature. In Chapter 3, you learned that the doshas exist in different proportions in each person. Some people may be predominantly Pitta, while others may have more Vata or Kapha. The dominant dosha can be balanced by eating or avoiding certain foods. For example, anyone with strong Pitta should avoid hot, spicy foods, as these will only increase Pitta's already concentrated influence.

During the first stage of disease, the doshas increase in mild amounts in their own seats—that is, the sites where they usually reside. Vata resides in the colon, Pitta in the small intestines, and Kapha in the stomach. The initial accumulation of the three doshas in the gastrointestinal tract can produce certain symptoms. When Vata begins to increase, your digestion might be erratic. If Pitta collects, you might feel a mild increase in body temperature. The buildup of Kapha might produce a feeling of heaviness.

These indications are mild, and most people don't pay any attention to them. Usually the body tries to counteract them early by craving foods that will balance the dosha that is increasing. For example, eating oily, heavy foods helps normalize Vata. If you are in tune with your body, you will follow its natural tendencies to balance itself. Most often, though, in today's busy world, people are not tuned in to their bodies' signals, or they won't take time to acknowledge them. They just keep eating the food or following the lifestyle that caused the imbalance in the first place. Consequently, the doshas continue to accrue until aggravation, the next stage of disease, develops.

Stage Two: Aggravation

In this stage of disease, the doshas continue to accumulate to the point where they become vitiated—spoiled or imbalanced. It's as if they become uncomfortable with remaining in their natural locations, and begin to develop a tendency to move to other locations in the body.

At this point, it is still relatively easy to make changes in diet or routine to keep the doshas in their homes in the digestive tract. However, some symptoms may still arise. For example, aggravated Vata can cause bloating or mild, pricking pain in the digestive tract. Or, it might produce excessive movement of materials in the digestive tract or increased contractions of the colon to move waste matter downward and out of the body. Vitiated Pitta generates a sour taste in the mouth, thirst, and a burning sensation inside the digestive tract or other places in the body. Aggravated Kapha can create nausea, an aversion to food, or pressure in the chest. These are important warning signs that should be heeded, but bear in mind that this stage of aggravation may be reached without any obvious symptoms whatsoever.

Stage Three: Dissemination

In this phase, instead of affecting their own domains, the doshas start to leave their primary seats in the digestive tract to travel to other sites in the body. Vata leaves the colon. Pitta leaves the small intestine. Kapha leaves the stomach. Initially, they tend to spread to the sites of their subdoshas. For example, Vata may travel to the head, throat, chest or circulatory system. Pitta could travel to the skin, blood, heart, or other sites. Kapha might move to the muscles, back, chest, and so forth. In a more advanced stage of dissemination, the doshas can move to sites governed by other doshas. Vata spreads to Pitta and Kapha sites, Pitta spreads to the seats of Kapha and Vata, and so on.

At this stage, too much exercise, too much hot, sharp food, and pressures that aggravate Vata can push the aggravated doshas into the srotas.

Vata is called the "king dosha" because it moves the other two. According to the Ayurvedic texts, "Vata, Pitta, and Kapha move in all the channels of the body, but due to subtleness, Vata provokes the other two doshas. Aggravated Vata excites Pitta and Kapha, and, carrying them to different places, it produces different disorders, such as obstruction in the passages and drying up of the dhatus, etc."[25] That is why Maharishi Vedic Medicine always takes precautions to keep Vata dosha in balance.

Like a river overflowing its banks, Vata floods into the areas governed by Pitta and Kapha, or Pitta overflows into places governed by Kapha and Vata, or Kapha into places governed by Vata and Pitta. This can result in a variety of symptoms. When Vata broadens its terrain, it can generate movement in the wrong direction or cause gurgling in the digestive tract. Pitta can cause a burning sensation in the digestive tract. Expanded Kapha can produce loss of taste or appetite, indigestion, weakness or tiredness in the body parts, and vomiting. At this stage, the symptoms are more powerful than before, and sometimes the person feels unhealthy enough to seek the help of a physician.

The doshas spread throughout the body during the aggravation and dissemination stages via two methods. First, Vata, the king dosha, spurs the increased Pitta and Kapha to move sites of the other doshas. Second the three doshas combine with the nutrient fluid, rasa dhatu, and circulate throughout the body. The doshas circulating through the nutritional fluid create a large range of symptoms related to Vata, Pitta, and Kapha. These range from pain in various parts of the body to tremors, improper digestion, and fainting.

Stage Four: Localization

Until this point in the disease process, the vitiated doshas have been circulating throughout the body via rasa dhatu. As the doshas accumulate due to unhealthy diet and behavior, agni (the digestive fire) becomes weaker and produces several unfortunate results. Ama, the waste product of abnormal digestion, forms and ojas diminishes. Abnormalities in the dhatus and blockage in the srotas also develop.

When abnormal doshas and ama mix with the nutritional fluid, they form a kind of sludge—a thick, sticky substance that is not nourishing to the tissues. It is so thick that it is actually incapable of entering into the minute channels that are designed to carry healthy nutritional fluid to the tissues. This sludge accumulates outside the tissue cells and causes the srotas and dhatus to swell.

This is how imbalanced doshas settle in specific places. It is also how they come in contact with tissues (dhatus) and normal waste products (malas), which by now are also imbalanced or distorted. When abnormal doshas and distorted dhatus and malas come together, this union of two or more abnormal substances creates great distress in the body.

The srotas are also involved in the degeneration process, because by now they are clogged, and the movement of rasa dhatu mixed with the doshas is obstructed. When blocked, the doshas become stagnant and begin to produce abnormal tissues. This becomes the location where the disease will manifest. However, at this point, specific diseases are still not identifiable.

Why does one srota become imbalanced rather than another? Abnormalities of the srotas are associated with decreased ojas. Consequently, a srota weakened by lack of ojas becomes the site where disease begins. Four influences debilitate the srotas: addictions, pollution, wrong routine and wrong food. All of these disrupt the intelligence of a particular area.

In this fourth stage, then, abnormalities are found in the doshas, dhatus, srotas, ojas, and agni, which leads to the localization of abnormalities and distress. The body expresses its distress in general symptoms—warning signals—like the whistle of an oncoming train.

Symptoms at this stage can resemble the indications of a specific disease, but usually they are more general. Based on the symptoms alone, it is difficult to accurately predict the future disease at this or any previous stage, which is why Maharishi Vedic Medicine does not rely on symptoms to diagnose.

By stage five, or manifestation, the disease is full-blown and much more difficult to cure. Unfortunately, most people do not consult their physicians until the disease is already far beyond the preventive period.

Stage Five: Manifestation

In Maharishi Vedic Medicine, people are not considered healthy if they are in any of the first four stages of disease, which they usually experience only as general feelings of discomfort or lack of ease. A physician trained in Maharishi Vedic Medicine can easily detect these early phases, however, by identifying imbalances in the doshas, dhatus, agni, and ojas through a number of sensitive techniques, including pulse diagnosis.

Unless the body is brought back into balance during the first four phases, the doshas and dhatus enter into the fifth stage of the disease process, in which fully developed symptoms show up. This stage is referred to as "clear manifestation," and "undoubtful appearance." Here the classic symptoms of disease are obvious and cause suffering. This is the phase that most Western medicine is geared to address. If you come to your medical doctor in the previous stages of disease and say, "I just don't feel right," he probably will not be able to pinpoint anything. He needs to see a recognizable symptom.

In Maharishi Vedic Medicine symptoms are classified as general—produced by increase in the doshas and found in all diseases—or specific to a particular disorder. Specific symptoms are produced not only by increased doshas, but also by abnormalities in the dhatus, srotas, and malas. General symptoms are more powerful, and are found all over the body. They are caused by unsuitable food and activity. Specific symptoms are fewer in number and are localized in only a few organs and places.

Since unsuitable diet and activity can constitute a chief source of an illness with general symptoms, the illness can sometimes be cured simply by adjusting diet and behavior to rebalance the doshas and strengthen agni and ojas. This removes the general cause of disease, and sometimes clears up the specific or localized symptoms as well. If not, the physician will prescribe measures to eliminate the root of the symptoms—abnormalities in the doshas, dhatus, and srotas. In any case, the physician will correct the imbalance at its source, rather than just treat its superficial indications.

Certain factors decrease the severity of illness. For example, the dominance of sattva in the mind increases mental strength and will-power. As a result, the disease is weaker and produces fewer, milder symptoms. In addition, when the dhatus and ojas are strong, symptoms are diminished and less severe.

At this stage of disease, it is still possible to cure the person with proper treatment. However, the treatment must be strong enough. If the treatment is only medium in strength, it pacifies the increased doshas to some extent but does not bring them completely into balance and back to their natural sites. This can create a situation where the doshas remain dormant in the tissues until a disturbance of some kind—either emotional or physical—activates them and they begin to increase again. In other words, if the treatment only aims to dissolve the symptoms but does not eradicate the fundamental source of disease, it may provide temporary relief, but the disease will surely recur.

Stage Six: Disruption

If the primary source of illness has not yet been eliminated, the doshas continue to increase and create damage. During the sixth stage, the abnormal changes that take place in the doshas, dhatus, and srotas are unpredictable, profound, greatly damaging, potentially chronic, and can even lead to death. The pores of the cells (srotas) become hard, rough, distorted, curved, irregular, closed shut, or constantly open. They lose or increase their functioning or develop hardness and growths.

Quite often, if strength and immunity (level of ojas) are weak, the individual experiences secondary complications. One disease actually creates the other. For example, if a person has a chronic, long-term cough, the disorder could spread into connecting areas and become asthma. If this individual is then exposed to tuberculosis and other organisms, he may develop a third disease, while a healthy person would remain immune. Chronic disease shatters the area where the intelligence of the body has been shadowed for a long time. If not corrected, the long-term disease starts shattering the coordination of intelligence in the whole body.

Secondary diseases are often caused by eating the same unsuitable foods and performing the same unsuitable activities that created the original disease. They can also be generated by inappropriate or ineffective medical treatment (iatrogenic disease). Individuals with strong ojas have a greater capacity to endure and withstand the effects of disease, and are far less likely to develop a secondary illness. Consequently, Maharishi Vedic Medicine always aims to increase ojas and physiological strength and never does anything that diminishes it.

Once the chronic phase of disease emerges, it is difficult to predict how the disease will spread. Think of this analogy that describes the intricacy of the human body: When you drive through the countryside, you see an environment composed of innumerable details—birds, animals, trees, rocks, grass, flowers, sky, clouds. It's a complex but beautiful picture. If a natural disaster such as a hurricane or tornado strikes, some parts of the landscape are destroyed immediately, while others manifest secondary effects later on. Some areas deteriorate quickly, and others take longer to degenerate. In the same way, when a disease becomes chronic within the complex landscape created by the myriad structures and functions of the human body, some areas are affected first, some later.

When disease spreads to more than one area of the body, it becomes more difficult to treat and produces more physiological deterioration. Even when disease settles in only one area, the distorted cells sometimes have to be surgically removed. If a disease keeps progressing sequentially, it becomes a multisystem disorder, affecting not just one organ, but many organs and systems. A person could have a headache, digestive problems, arthritis and fatigue all at once. Such complications are increasingly hard to diagnose and treat. Disease can also become incurable. That is why we always stress prevention.

There is a story about a king who had many wise counselors and great wealth and fame, but never took care of himself. His ministers warned him that he needed to pay more attention to his body, to rest more, to eat healthier foods, and to follow the seasonal routines. He continued to lead an unhealthy lifestyle, foolishly declaring that if he ever fell ill he could simply hire the best physicians and buy the best medicines. When symptoms arose, he used band-aid type cures to fix his health problems, without addressing the cause—his unhealthy lifestyle.

Eventually, due to continued poor diet and routine, he developed a chronic disease. By the time he called a physician, it had already become incurable. The king then put out a flyer promising to give half his kingdom to anyone who could cure him. Unfortunately, no amount of money could buy back his good health. He had waited too long. The foolish king did not act to prevent and treat his disease early enough to save himself.

As disease gets complicated and involves imbalances in all the doshas, diagnosis and treatment also become complicated. If all three doshas are highly aggravated, it becomes difficult to determine which to bring into balance first. When you catch illness early enough, it is easier to recognize localized and specific causes.

In my practice, I have observed that chronic disease does not exist as a separate entity, and that curing a symptom does not necessarily mean you've cured the disease. Until all six stages of disease have been redressed, the patient cannot be declared cured. In conventional medical textbooks, every chronic disease is listed as one illness, such as chronic asthma, chronic hypertension, or chronic arthritis.

However, only rarely do patients have just one illness. Most of the time doctors find an associated disease and group of symptoms. For example, a hypertension patient may have headaches and associated digestive problems, depression and associated arthritis. Similarly, a patient with digestive problems may have chronic fatigue or menstrual disorders.

Because conventional doctors see every illness as separate and relate illness to a group of organs, they target only the symptoms in devising treatment. Medical specialization was created because of this, and many specialists are just now realizing we must treat the whole person. I believe that in a few years, every physician will be aware of Maharishi Vedic Medicine. Soon thereafter, I hope, every physician will begin using it to treat and prevent chronic disease, because without this holistic approach, there is no hope for conquering chronic disease.

An Illustration of the Six Stages of Disease

Imagine that one spring morning two men each buy identical new cars. Their cars both operate smoothly and bring them a lot of enjoyment. Five years later, Bob's car still operates well, much as it did when he first bought it. Larry's car, on the other hand, is in the junkyard.

What went wrong with Larry's car? Let's go back to the day the men first bought the cars. Bob changed the oil after every 3,000 miles and serviced his car regularly. Larry, on the other hand, never changed his oil. Let's look at the stages of the demise of Larry's car over the five years.

Stage 1: Accumulation. Since Larry has not changed the oil, the old oil starts to accumulate dust and dirt.

Stage 2: Aggravation. Dust and dirt, which should have been removed from the car by replacing the oil every 3,000 miles, permeates the oil.

Stage 3: Dissemination. Dirt begins to circulate throughout the entire engine. At this stage, Larry's car still runs without any problems. While a skilled mechanic would be able to tell the difference in the engine (it wouldn't run as smoothly as before), most people would see no outward signs of dirt in the oil.

Stage 4: Localization. The dirty oil, which was circulating throughout the engine, now gets so thick that it can no longer pass easily through the screen that protects the oil pump. Less and less oil passes through the screen, and thus less and less oil gets pumped through the engine. For the first time, the engine begins to cough a little, and Larry notices there is a slight loss of power at certain times when he is operating his vehicle. The valve lifters start to make a ticking noise, since there is not enough oil lubricating them. Larry ignores these symptoms. He doesn't know exactly what is wrong, but he knows the engine is showing vague signs of problems.

Stage 5: Manifestation. Now Larry has trouble starting the car. The oil has become a thick sludge, and very little oil can pass through the screen and get pumped into the engine. Even when the car starts, friction in the pistons causes loud knocking and the steering wheel starts vibrating violently. Larry knows something is wrong, but keeps driving until he can reach a gas station.

Stage 6: Disruption. Larry notices black smoke pouring out of the engine. The car quits on the highway and has to be towed to the repair shop. From lack of clean oil, the pistons froze, the bearings wore out, and the camshaft broke. When Larry goes to pick up his car, the mechanic tells him that his car now rests in the junkyard.

This problem did not happen suddenly. Larry thought his vehicle ran normally during stages 1, 2, and 3, but in fact things started to go wrong with the engine's operation before any symptoms appeared. In this analogy, Western medicine would try and treat the symptoms—give Larry's car new pistons, valve lifters, and bearings. However, unless the root of the problem—dirty oil—is addressed, the car's symptoms will reappear and continue. And it's so much easier to change the oil!

Maharishi Vedic Medicine identifies disease at an early stage and eliminates its primary source, thus preventing the development of symptoms. In cases where symptoms have already manifested, the main focus is still removal of the fundamental cause. Once the cause is dissolved, symptoms automatically disappear.

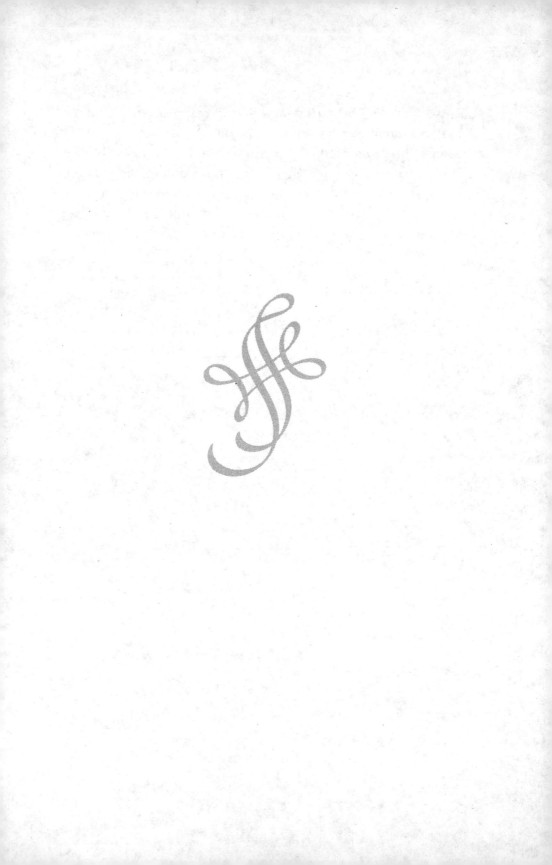

CHAPTER 10

Arthritis and Asthma: Two Examples of the Development of Chronic Disease

"It is in the interest of everyone, healthy or otherwise, to own this knowledge of the total range of health— from individual to cosmic—to maintain balance in life, the basis of good health."   —*Maharishi Mahesh Yogi*[26]

Now that you have seen how a disorder can start with a doshic imbalance and progress into life-threatening symptoms, here are two examples showing how a chronic disease develops.

Arthritis

Although most people think of swollen, painful joints when they say the word arthritis, modern medicine actually identifies nearly 100 types of arthritis. Two common types are osteoarthritis and rheumatoid arthritis.

Osteoarthritis is perhaps the most common form of arthritis in people who are past middle age. It usually begins as a result of wear and tear on the joints during the latter part of life, and is characterized by a degenerative process in the joints. For example, cartilage softens and erodes and the affected joints swell, becoming stiff and painful. Even though all the joints of the body are vulnerable, the weight-bearing joints, such as the knee and elbow, are most commonly involved. In the elderly, the disease frequently attacks the hip and shoulder joints.

Rheumatoid Arthritis from a Modern Medical Perspective

Rheumatoid arthritis is more serious because it is an autoimmune disease that can cause inflammation of the joints and other organs of the body, including the glands of the eyes and mouth and the lining of the heart and lungs. Rheumatoid arthritis affects approximately 2.1 million people in the United States (one per cent of the general population). It strikes people of all ages, although the average age is 30 to 40. Three times more women than men are affected in the 20-to-50 year age group, although after age 50 the disease occurs equally in men and women.[27]

Common symptoms include fatigue; low-grade fever; loss of appetite and weight; morning joint stiffness; pain, swelling, and inflammation in the finger joints, wrists, and feet; nodules forming near affected joints; and joint deformities. There is no known cause of rheumatoid arthritis, and it is now considered to be an autoimmune disease, meaning that the immune system starts attacking itself, as in the case of AIDS. According to one theory, certain individuals have a weak immune system, making them genetically susceptible to a virus that attacks the joints.

Modern Medical Treatments of
Rheumatoid Arthritis and Their Side Effects

Although ten per cent of people with rheumatoid arthritis experience a spontaneous remission, many others are faced with pain and disabling joint deformity. The treatments include four powerful drugs: nonsteroidal anti-inflammatory drugs (NSAIDs) to reduce swelling and pain; corticosteroids, which are more effective in treating swelling and pain but with more serious side effects; disease-modifying antirheumatic drugs (DMARDs), slower-acting drugs that may bring about a temporary remission and inhibit degeneration and deformity of the joint; and immunosuppressive drugs, which are used only in extreme cases because side effects are severe.

Side effects include nausea, gastrointestinal tract irritation and bleeding, rashes, ulcers, and impaired renal function for NSAIDs. Weight gain, puffy face, thinning of the skin and bone, tendency to bruise easily, severe mood swings, and insomnia for corticosteroids. Skin rash, nausea and vomiting, diarrhea, anemia, muscle weakness, and kidney and bone marrow damage for DMARDs. Depressed bone marrow functioning, low white blood cell count, cirrhosis of the liver, and allergic reactions in the lungs for immunosuppressive drugs.[28]

The Cause of Arthritis from the Perspective of Maharishi Vedic Medicine

Arthritis is a systemic disease. This means that it involves whole systems of the body, and is not just located where the symptoms appear in the joints, as many people believe. In addition to the many signs and symptoms described, arthritis patients also suffer from various disorders in different parts of the body. They often complain of chronic digestive disorders, chronic constipation, general fatigue, emotional stress, lack of sufficient rest, nutritional deficiencies, hormonal and endocrine disorders, and other dysfunctions. These symptoms occur long before the final symptoms appear in the joints. It is important to understand that if arthritis is to be successfully treated, the physician must follow a holistic approach and recognize not only the systemic nature of the disease and its abnormal conditions, but he or she must recognize the disorders in other parts of the body that need to be corrected as well.

Arthritis is a chronic disease. Its most common symptom is pain in the joints. At first, it may be slow or low-intensity pain, and the patient may experience difficulty in climbing stairs and lifting heavy objects. The pain may come and go and disappear in response to pain killers, or it may subside with just a little rest. Sometimes it disappears for months at a time and then reappears. There may be stiffness and numbness of the joints, the joints may crack, and they often become swollen and inflamed. In the early stages, pain can be mild or acute, or largely appear in the morning or at night. The pain may be aggravated by exposure to cold, wind or rain.

The current treatment of arthritis suppresses the pain and relieves the inflammation or swelling. This, however, gives a false sense of relief to the patient. It is dangerous because the disease continues to progress inside the body, and at one stage or another, both the patient and the physician become helpless. The patient cannot use his joints, and the physician cannot reduce the pain or swelling and provide relief, let alone arrest the progress of the disease.

It's important to note that the appearance of pain or joint stiffness is not the first stage of the disease, it is actually the fourth stage. It has become a systemic disorder. Without the person being aware of it, toxins have been accumulating in the blood and joints for a long time before the first signal of approaching arthritis was experienced in the form of joint pain. The patient has usually abused his or her body for years through wrong diet, unhealthy lifestyle, physical and mental stress, and insufficient rest to produce the level of doshic disturbance that leads to the breakdown of health and joint function.

Vata, Pitta, and Kapha, when out of balance, all have a role in rheumatoid arthritis, but Maharishi Vedic Medicine identifies vitiated Vata as the main aggravating factor. Vata regulates the nervous system and all movement in the body, and governs all sensory and motor activities. In osteoarthritis aggravated Vata is associated with ama, a product of improper digestion. Consequently, the treatment for either form of arthritis includes alleviation of

Vata, plus correction of other imbalances and correction of ama formation.

Aggravation of the Doshas

In a healthy person, the three doshas are normally in a state of homeostasis, or equilibrium. Usually the body tolerates some changes in the equilibrium, but when the doshas become imbalanced, sickness can begin. Arthritis starts with vitiated Vata. However, the fluid in the synovial membrane of the joints is regulated by Kapha. The metabolic by-products of abnormal digestion, such as ama, are the outcome of Pitta activity. Thus all three doshas, when out of balance, are separately or jointly involved in producing arthritis.

Vata normally gets aggravated during the dry, windy season. A number of other factors also derange Vata, including excessive exercise, fasting, a fall or an injury, sleep disorders, suppression of natural urges, suppression of worries or stress, exposure to cold, facing fearful situations, and the long-term intake of foods that are pungent, dry, astringent, or bitter.

Cold generally deranges Vata and Kapha and also impairs the functioning of Pitta. Impaired Pitta functioning affects digestive and metabolic processes. Undesirable metabolic by-products—ama and free radicals which feed on ama—are created. These imbalances, coupled with abnormal metabolic by-products, produce or intensify arthritis if not corrected for a long period. This intensification is particularly seen in the winter and rainy season, or when there is more humidity or relatively low temperatures.

Blocked Srotas and Dhatu Deterioration

If the vitiated doshas are not corrected through diet and lifestyle changes, the dhatus (tissues) start to get distorted. The tissues involved in the joints include the ligaments, synovial fluid, tissue cells, tendons, and muscles. The ends of the bones are covered with an elastic tissue called cartilage, and synovial membrane covers the inner surfaces of the joint cavities. This membrane secretes a fluid that lubricates the joints.

The synovial membrane and the tips of the bones are provided with several capillaries that carry nourishment along with blood to the joints. If any infections, toxins, or incomplete metabolic by-products pass through these capillaries (srotas), the circulation of the nutrients and blood is obstructed. The result is stagnation and exudation in the pocket created by the synovial membrane of the joint; that is, unwanted fluids such as serum, blood, or pus flow into the joint.

The joint becomes inflamed, enlarged, and swollen. Due to improper nourishment, the cartilage loses its elasticity and becomes dry and brittle, and secretion of the synovial membrane also diminishes. The joint dries out and grows congested and stiff. This may also cause the surrounding ligaments and tendons to become inflamed and progressively to lose their tone and flexibility. As a consequence of faulty metabolism and movement, excessive amounts of calcium and other minerals are deposited in the joints. In some cases, osteoporosis, or leaching of calcium and other minerals from the bones, causes serious destruction of the bones and joints.

All these changes are usually accompanied by swelling and pain during movement. Subsequently the person becomes incapable of moving the affected part of the body. If this development is not checked and treated in time, complete destruction of the joint and impairment of its function will often occur.

An Example of Arthritis Treatment with Maharishi Vedic Medicine

At 68, Eileen was diagnosed with rheumatoid arthritis. She complained of stiffness in her joints and pain in her shoulders and arms. Her primary care physician prescribed Prednizone but with little relief. She had trouble sleeping at night, and suffered from frequent sinus problems.

Her treatments from Maharishi Vedic Medicine included herbal formulas, a special diet to balance her doshas, an herbalized oil treatment for the nasal passages, and changes in her daily routine, such as daily Ayurvedic oil massage. She also learned the Transcendental Meditation technique to help relieve stress and activate her body's natural healing system. She was soon able to cut back on the Prednizone as some of the symptoms subsided.

"I began to feel more energetic," she said. "I did everything faithfully, and it helped. I especially enjoyed the oil massage every morning. It was very relaxing and helped soothe the joints. Doing the Transcendental Meditation technique also helped me reduce stress, and gave me the deep rest I needed to fight this disease. I've found that these approaches treat the cause, rather than the symptoms. The herbal formulas and other therapies helped strengthen the immune system to fight this autoimmune disease. The treatments seemed to address my whole system. I've had no sinus problems since I started the treatments."

Asthma

Asthma is a chronic lung disease that affects nearly six per cent of the population. It can occur any time in a person's life, starting from infancy. Asthma is now on the rise, especially among children. The last decade has seen a 50 per cent increase in doctor's visits due to asthma.

A person with asthma often suffers from attacks of shortness of breath, tightness of the chest, wheezing, forced breathing, and coughing. The person usually has trouble exhaling. Other possible symptoms include spasms or tightness in the muscles surrounding the bronchial tubes, swelling of the bronchial tube lining, constriction of the airways, and production of large amounts of mucus.

There are several types of asthma:

Extrinsic asthma, caused by allergens such as dust, dust mites, pollens, animal danders, feathers, wool, and molds.

Intrinsic asthma, caused by an unusual and specific sensitivity to a particular substance.

Occupational asthma, caused by irritating chemicals or dust on the job.

Exercise-induced asthma, which usually occurs only in children and young adults.[29]

The Cause of Asthma from the Perspective of Modern Medicine

Allergens such as animal fur, dust, dander, mold, and pollen can trigger asthma, as can emotional stress and exercise. Heredity, exposure to cigarette smoke, and certain medications (aspirin, sleeping pills, and drugs for blood pressure and heart) can also cause asthma.

Modern Medical Treatments of Asthma and Their Side Effects

According to Western medical practice, asthma is a response to certain allergens and triggers, and can be eliminated if these triggers are avoided. However, in Western medical practice, nonallergic forms of asthma are usually not considered curable. Medications aim to manage the disease by providing relief from acute asthmatic attacks, stabilizing lung function, preventing recurrent acute attacks, and preventing later complications such as emphysema or heart disease. Physicians usually prescribe two kinds of asthma medications—anti-inflammatory drugs, which are designed to prevent asthma attacks, and bronchodilators, which are inhaled as sprays and help bring relief during an attack.

The most common side effects of bronchodilators are headache, muscle tremor, heartburn, heart palpitations, elevated blood pressure, nausea, nervousness, and dizziness. Anti-inflammatory drugs create side effects such as hoarseness or loss of voice, bruising, yeast infection, altered bone density and adrenal suppression.

Non-drug treatments include removing dust and mites from living areas, using air filters in home heating and cooling systems, avoiding cigarette smoke, and avoiding irritants and chemicals on the job.

The Cause of Asthma from the Perspective of Maharishi Vedic Medicine

The Ayurvedic texts identify five types of asthma: *kshudra* (simple or mild), *tamaka* (pertaining to darkness), *chhinna* (interrupted), *urddha* (upward), and *maha* (severe or grave). Kshudra is the most common type, and it is the type Western physicians identify as asthma. The others occur only rarely and are more severe.

Aggravating Factors Identified by Maharishi Vedic Medicine

- Eating foods that aggravate Kapha and Vata (very rich, heavy, dry, cold)
- Residence in cold places
- Exposure to smoke, dust or allergens, which irritate the nose and respiratory passages
- Exposure to sun or strong wind
- Heavy or violent exercise; carrying heavy loads; long, tiring walks and exercise
- Suppression of natural urges
- Fasting

When disease manifests, it does so in a particular organ, but does not necessarily originate from that organ. Maharishi Vedic Medicine describes three different pathological arenas: the site of disease origin, the channels of circulation, and the site of disease manifestation. It's important to understand that in the case of asthma, the disease actually starts in the gastrointestinal system and then localizes in the lungs.

The stomach and colon, the seats of Kapha and Vata, are the sites at which asthma begins. Ama (pathogenic substance) behind the manifestation of this disease originates from these places. Ama travels from the site of origin through a group of channels called *rasavaha srotas.* Rasavaha srotas are the channels that carry the nourishing fluids (rasa) from the intestines to the tissues. They also remove excreted waste products from these tissues and carry the wastes to the different channels of elimination: rectum, urinary bladder, and so on.

When digestion is disturbed through wrong diet, lifestyle, or routine, ama starts to collect. It mixes with rasa, and the rasavaha srotas start transporting these pathogenic substances to other parts of the body—in the case of asthma, to the lungs.

Once ama is created, due to disturbances in the stomach and gastrointestinal tract and aggravated Kapha, the agnis also get disturbed. The agnis govern the enzymes in the gastrointestinal tract, liver, and tissues. Consequently, digestion and metabolism are disrupted and much of the resulting unhealthy end-product of incomplete digestion (ama) accumulates in the intestines, the liver, and the bloodstream. When there is improper digestion and metabolism—at the gastrointestinal level, in the liver, and at the tissue level—ama is the result.

The Site of Manifestation

When ama circulates in the blood it forms an impure nutritive fluid called ama-rasa. The ama-rasa travels to the lungs, where it causes obstruction of the bronchial tubes and of the blood vessels in the *alveoli* (the little air sacs where oxygen is absorbed into the blood). This produces spasms or contractions, which are asthmatic symptoms.

When the ama-rasa settles in the lungs, Vata and Kapha become excited and obstruct the respiratory ducts of the body. These ducts carry the life-breath, known as the upward-moving subdoshas of Vata, *Prana* and *Udana*. Vata itself, obstructed by Kapha, is turned from its normal course to other directions, producing difficult breathing, spasms, and coughing.[30]

The Deeper Causes of Asthma

Maharishi Vedic Medicine does not see allergens as the cause of asthma. Irritating substances are always floating in the air, yet not everyone who inhales them becomes ill. Only a few individuals suffer from asthma, and those who do have some weakness in their lungs. In these individuals, the lung tissue, the tissues and musculature of the bronchial tubes, and the mucous membrane linings of these tubes are enervated, producing less ojas.

In the case of asthma, any ama produced by the body travels to the lungs because the lungs are a vulnerable point in that patient's body.

What creates this weak point? Excessive use or wrong use of that part of the physiology causes dosha accumulation. For example, people who smoke are more susceptible to asthma. Seasonal effects can also tax the body. In Kapha season, for example, ama tends to collect in the lungs. A weak area can also be inherited.

Wrong diet, daily and seasonal routines, medicines, psychological factors, and certain climatic conditions such as damp, cold weather, can all precipitate asthma because they throw the doshas out of equilibrium and contribute to the production of ama.

One of the principles of treatment in Maharishi Vedic Medicine is to strengthen the vulnerable spot in the body to avoid disease. The weak area is the main cause of localization of disease, and if it is aggravated, the illness is more likely to start.

In asthma, the sensitive area is the lungs, and in arthritis, it is the joints. In other conditions, the weak spot might be the heart or blood. By strengthening the immune system and the body's sensitive points, and by improving the end-products of digestion so that ama is reduced, the disease process is far less likely to be triggered.

An Example of Asthma Treatment with Maharishi Vedic Medicine

Theresa, a 71-year-old secretary for the New York State Assembly, suffered from such severe bouts of bronchitis-induced asthma that she had to be hospitalized every three months like clockwork.

She feels her asthma, allergies, and bronchitis were aggravated by pollutants in her workplace. "I know the building I work in is very unhealthy," she said. "It was built on a landfill, and the building is new—only seven years old. My asthma attacks began six years ago."

Her last attack, like the others, started with bronchitis. Her doctor gave her antibiotics and Prednizone. Sensing that this attack was more severe, he advised her to go to the hospital, but she thought she'd wait it out. She ended up in the emergency room fearing for her life.

After her brush with death, she decided to get to the bottom of her illness. She told her doctor she didn't want to continue with allergy shots. "I am tired of putting chemicals into my system," she told her doctor. "This is like putting band-aids on." In the meantime, an acquaintance told her about Maharishi Vedic Medicine, and she decided to give it a try, with the wholehearted support of her primary physician. Just nine months later, Theresa is off every single Western medication. She no longer suffers from bronchitis every three months and has not had a single asthmatic attack.

"I feel better than I have felt in years," she said. "My allergies are better, too. I haven't even had the sinus infections or headaches. Just a couple of sneezy days, but nothing I can't handle. I am amazed. I had no idea how phenomenal it would be. I am not exaggerating, it really has been a miracle."

Theresa's treatments included the Transcendental Meditation technique to reduce mental and physical stress and balance the entire mind-body system, Vedic breathing exercises to strengthen and purify her lungs, Maharishi Ayur-Veda herbal supplements to improve immunity and strengthen her lungs, dietary recommendations to balance the doshas, and a special therapy called *nasya* which purifies and strengthens the nasal passages and lungs.

"The best thing is, I'm not putting anything harmful in my system," says Theresa. "Occasionally I do have to use the Ventilin® spray, but gradually I'm getting weaned off that, too. It has taken a while to purify my body of all the drugs I was on before. Even my general practitioner is impressed. He said, 'Do you realize you haven't had an emergency in a year? It's absolutely amazing.'"

Research on Maharishi Vedic Medicine and Asthma

Dramatic improvements have been found in patients with bronchial asthma who practice the Transcendental Meditation technique, one of the primary approaches of Maharishi Vedic Medicine. Patients in one study exhibited decreased severity of symptoms, including reduced airway resistance.

This chapter has focused on the details of the progression of two chronic diseases. However, it is important not to lose sight of the main purpose of Maharishi Vedic Medicine—to create wholeness, or ideal health. While illness can localize in one specific area—such as joints, in arthritis—Maharishi Vedic Medicine recognizes that the localized disease is not the primary problem. The fundamental problem is that the diseased area of the body has lost its alignment with the body's underlying intelligence. The solution is to reconnect that area with Nature's pure intelligence and perfect orderliness so that it functions in perfect relationship to the whole physiology. Treatments can include diet, Maharishi Yoga℠ postures (*asanas*), herbal preparations, rejuvenation therapies, or dozens of other approaches. All the therapeutic modalities have one common objective: Eliminate the obstacles to the flow of healing intelligence. Then the whole mind-body can move in the direction of bliss and eventually reach the goal of enlightenment,

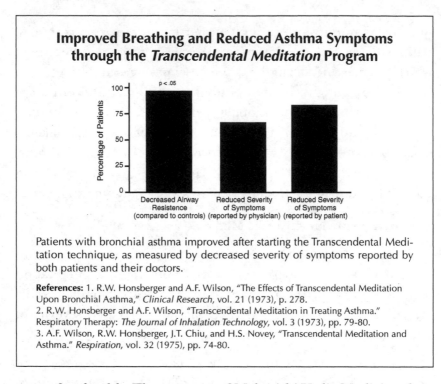

Improved Breathing and Reduced Asthma Symptoms through the *Transcendental Meditation* Program

Patients with bronchial asthma improved after starting the Transcendental Meditation technique, as measured by decreased severity of symptoms reported by both patients and their doctors.

References: 1. R.W. Honsberger and A.F. Wilson, "The Effects of Transcendental Meditation Upon Bronchial Asthma," *Clinical Research*, vol. 21 (1973), p. 278.
2. R.W. Honsberger and A.F. Wilson, "Transcendental Meditation in Treating Asthma." Respiratory Therapy: *The Journal of Inhalation Technology*, vol. 3 (1973), pp. 79-80.
3. A.F. Wilson, R.W. Honsberger, J.T. Chiu, and H.S. Novey, "Transcendental Meditation and Asthma." *Respiration*, vol. 32 (1975), pp. 74-80.

or perfect health. The purpose of Maharishi Vedic Medicine does not stop with eliminating illnesses such as arthritis or asthma—that is only a by-product of the ultimate goal of bringing all aspects of the individual body and mind in alignment with the healing power of Nature.

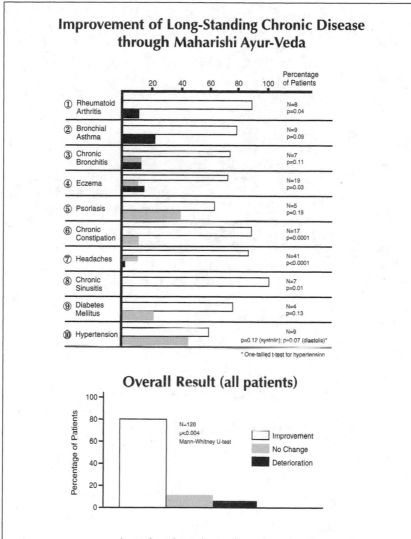

Improvement of Long-Standing Chronic Disease through Maharishi Ayur-Veda

In a more recent study, Maharishi Vedic Medicine brought substantial improvement in seven out of ten chronic diseases—including bronchial asthma—in a short period of time.

Reference: G.W.H.M. Janssen, "The Maharishi Ayur-Vedic Treatment of Ten Chronic Diseases: A Pilot Study." *Nederlands Tijdschrift voor Intergratie Geneeskunde*, vol. 5, (1989), pp. 56-94.

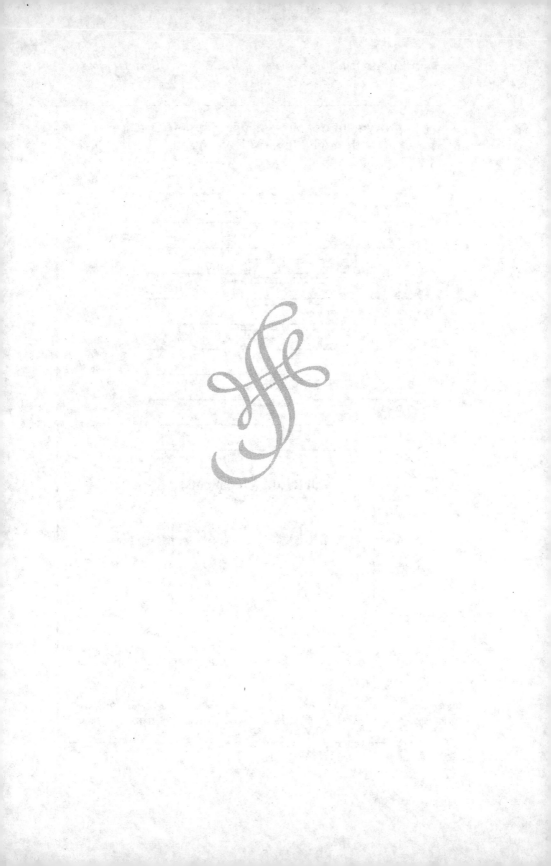

PART IV
The Road Back to Health

The Road Back to Health

The previous sections introduced the important perspective that Maharishi Vedic Medicine provides on the cause and progression of disease. Turning to happier matters, in this section you will discover the many ways in which the path to disease can be changed into a highway to health.

The following fifteen chapters will show how illness can be swept away by applying powerful treatments and therapies that focus on restoring wholeness and balance to the mind, body, emotions, behavior, and environment. The next chapters will detail the stages of treatment, the diagnostic procedures, and the full range of therapies used in Maharishi Vedic Medicine. These include therapies for restoring balance through diet and improved digestion, herbal supplements, daily routine, seasonal routine, sound therapy, rejuvenation therapy, therapies to harness the healing powers of the mind, and therapies to eliminate negative effects from the environment.

These modalities reflect a new vision for the treatment of chronic disease—a vision of health and wholeness. Their common focus is to enliven the body's inner healing intelligence, thereby allowing the body to repair itself. They restore health at the most fundamental level of the mind-body instead of just focusing on the diseased area. Where most treatments in modern medicine carry with them inevitable side effects, the treatments of Maharishi Vedic Medicine create side *benefits*, rejuvenating the mind and body in ways you never imagined possible.

CHAPTER 11

Undoing the Damage

"Maharishi's Vedic Approach to Health proceeds on
the road of balance between the holistic and specific
values of Natural Law. It starts from any level of imbalance and, eliminating imbalance, arrives at the level of
balance—integration of mind, body, behavior and
environment." —*Maharishi Mahesh Yogi*[31]

For someone who is very ill, it may seem difficult to take steps
to get well. It may even seem impossible. To encourage my patients to summon the courage to take the first step, I use the window analogy, to which I referred earlier in the book. When a
clean window collects dust, the view through the window gets
fuzzy. As the window collects more and more dust, you eventually
stop noticing that it is dirty at all. You become accustomed to seeing through a thick layer of dust. Then one morning, you clean
one small spot and discover just how dirty the window is. Perhaps
you don't have the energy to keep cleaning, because the job looks
overwhelming. However, you clean a little more the next day and
the next, and eventually the entire window is crystal clear.

Once the window is spotless, you notice the contrast when a
little layer of dust settles on it. Before, when the window was covered with grime, additional layers of dust could collect and you
wouldn't even notice. Now you notice even a thin layer of dust on
the window, and you can keep it clean with very little effort—just
a light dusting and it's done.

In the same way, you sometimes forget how important it is to take care of your body and you allow its functioning to deteriorate over time. You may not even recognize what's going on. It may happen so gradually that you don't notice your quality of life declining, until one day you get a wake-up call in the form of pain, physical malfunctioning or debilitation.

Once you start to reverse the damage through the therapies of Maharishi Vedic Medicine, you gradually restore your body to its natural state of balance. Then if the body starts accumulating imbalances again, you will notice immediately that something is wrong and take steps to correct it. The heightened sensitivity to your body's needs, which develops as your health improves, is the key to experiencing wellness and happiness each day of your life. Once you realize how little it takes to feel good you'll be less likely to fall back into old, health-destructive habits.

One of my patients, Jane, spoke to me once about this experience. When she was ill, Jane told me, she felt bad almost every day. Now that she has regained her health, when she has an "off" day she can hardly stand it. "I don't know how I tolerated feeling miserable for so long," she said. "Now I can bring myself back to normal readily, whereas I could not do that before."

The Limited Value of Symptomatic Treatment

The main focus of Maharishi Vedic Medicine is to restore the full expression of the body's inner intelligence and to correct physiological imbalances. In contrast, allopathic medicine centers on the diagnosis and treatment of disease symptoms. Trying to treat disease by focusing on symptoms is not very effective. Unless you eliminate the cause of the disease, as well as repair the physiological havoc it has wrought, the problem will surely recur—and not necessarily in the same location where the disorder first appeared.

A Definition of Health, Disease, and Treatment

Health is *swasthya*: permanent unfoldment of the deepest nature of the Self. In this state, the individual is fully attuned to Natural Law, the intelligence that upholds all evolution in Nature. He or she spontaneously functions in harmony with the inherent intelligence that governs the functioning of the doshas, dhatus, agni, srotas, mind, and senses.

Disease is a disruption in the flow of Natural Law, a breakdown in the sequential unfoldment of the body's inner intelligence. It can manifest as a lack of connection between organ tissue and body, or as a disturbance in the communication between organs and cellular tissues.

Treatment reestablishes the connection between the diseased organ's intelligence and the wholeness of the body's inner intelligence. Each cell starts to function in harmony with the part of the body to which it belongs, as well as with the totality of the body's inner intelligence.

Applying a band-aid treatment to stop symptoms generally does little to eliminate the cause and stop the progression of illness. At best, it buys some time, during which the body's own self-regulating intelligence may take care of the problem. At worst, it causes the problem to lodge even deeper in the physiology, and it may even create disorders of its own through the damage produced by drugs and toxic treatments. Drugs designed to knock out symptoms in one part of the body often create severe imbalances in other parts of the body. Drugs aim to destroy disease, not to strengthen the body's own ability to fight it. The result of this fragmented approach is damaged body tissue, weakened immunity and the creation of new disorders caused by the medicines themselves.

Of course, in some cases symptoms are so severe and dangerous that they need to be addressed immediately. However, this does not change the fact that it is far more effective to diagnose and treat an imbalance long before the symptoms arise.

A classic example of ineffective, symptom-based therapy can be found in the handling of hyperacidity. Western medicine often prescribes antacids for excess stomach acidity. While this may temporarily decrease stomach acidity and stop the burning sensation, it does nothing to address the hyperacidity's underlying source.

Maharishi Vedic Medicine takes a different approach. In talking with the patient, the physician might discover that his condition is linked to a habit of eating again before the previous meal is digested. This habit is quite common in our society, and unfortunately severely disrupts digestion. In an attempt to process new food, acids pour into the stomach, interfering with metabolism of the previously ingested food. The result is hyperacidity. On the surface, the problem appears linked to excess Pitta in the stomach—that is, acidity, heat and fire. However, this condition is really the product of an imbalance in the digestive fire which arose because of the patient's long-standing habit of eating at the wrong time. The solution is to strengthen digestion, not block it with antacids.

The Maharishi Vedic Medicine physician would advise this individual to prevent the problem by waiting at least three hours after a meal before eating again. If even then the prior meal is not yet fully digested, he should eat only light, liquid food to avoid overburdening the digestive system—and then only if really necessary. We might also recommend some digestive aids such as mild spices to increase the digestive fire. This is diametrically opposed to the Western prescription of antacids to decrease acidity!

Of course, hyperacidity can also have many other causes. To be permanently eliminated, it should be thoroughly diagnosed and properly treated by physicians trained in Maharishi Vedic Medicine.

One of the best things you can do to restore health to your digestive system and thereby improve your overall health, is to follow this simple principle: Don't eat again before the previous meal has been completely digested. How do you know when digestion is complete? It's simple. You feel hungry. Unfortunately, the eating habits of many people in our society are so aberrant that they rarely experience hunger between meals. The result is obesity and all sorts of long-term digestive disorders. If people could correct just this one behavior, it would drastically improve their vitality and well-being.

From Side Effects to Side Benefits

The therapies of Maharishi Vedic Medicine are natural and gentle. They work simultaneously to restore balance in both mind and body and to trigger the body's internal healing systems. Each treatment enlivens and renews the whole person—consciousness, mind, emotions, body, and environment.

Diet, for example, is used not only as a therapy to eliminate imbalances and restore health, but also to energize the flow of positive emotions and create greater clarity of mind. Eating the right foods with the right tastes balances the three doshas and creates greater physiological equilibrium and well-being. Consuming foods that are easy to digest helps the body eliminate toxins that can block the flow of inner intelligence and interfere with the full expression of your mental capacity. Finally, eating sattvic foods increases the level of ojas in the mind-body, boosting immunity, health, and happiness.

Ayurvedic oil massage is another treatment that affects mind, body and emotions. It strengthens muscles, enlivens the skin, eliminates toxins, and creates endorphins and immuno-modulators, which enhance immunity and create a sense of well-being. It also balances the doshas, creates ojas and opens the srotas.

Maharishi Ayur-Veda herbal formulas correct imbalances, reduce ama, and eliminate symptoms. Even though the herbal compounds are targeted at specific imbalances, each formula triggers the body's inner intelligence and enhances both mind and body.

A Step-by-Step, Yet All-in-One, Approach to Health

Just as Maharishi Vedic Medicine presents a sequential model for the development of disease, its treatment approaches are also sequential. The steps of treatment include:

- **Diagnose** the fundamental cause of illness.
- **Correct** pragya-aparadh, the first cause of all disorders.
- **Enliven** the body's inner intelligence so that the body can employ its powerful healing system to repair itself.
- **Correct** imbalances in the doshas, the mind-body operators.
- **Eliminate** ama (toxins and free radicals).
- **Build** dhatus. Repair damaged or depleted body tissues.
- **Open** the srotas, the channels of communication, nourishment, and waste removal.
- **Create** ojas, improving immunity and overall well-being.
- **Eliminate** symptoms.

You will note that eliminating symptoms is the last stage of treatment. Symptoms represent the last and most superficial manifestation of illness, the result of much deeper disturbances. Consequently, removal of symptoms is not the target of the treatments, but their automatic result.

As pointed out earlier, in Maharishi Vedic Medicine, *all* the therapies perform *all* the steps for recovery. Together they create a whole that is more than the sum of the parts, and they rejuvenate the entire mind-body system, not just the diseased area. This rejuvenation begins with the very first treatment, which is why the relief from distress is so remarkable right from the start. In the following chapters, you will see how each of these natural approaches helps undo the damage from chronic disease.

How the Treatments Worked Together to Create Health

Carrie was only 24 when she developed chronic asthma. A professional opera singer, she was under great stress when her asthma first appeared. She managed to get by for years by simply ignoring her problem. However, in her early thirties she came down with a life-threatening asthma attack and wound up in the hospital. After that experience, she went to a specialist who put her on steroids and other medications.

Heart disease ran in Carrie's family, so she was concerned about the side effects of some of her medications. They caused her heart to race and impaired liver functioning. To prevent asthma attacks, she took an anti-inflammatory, inhaled drug called Tilade three times a day; a steroid, Abuterol, four times a day; and an inhaled steroid four times a day. Despite these strong prescriptions, her asthma still flared up. No wonder Carrie started looking for alternative ways to heal herself.

Three years ago she read about the Transcendental Meditation technique and resolved to give it a try. Encouraged by the results, she decided to sign up for a week-long, in-residence stay at The Raj Maharishi Ayur-Veda Health Center in Fairfield, Iowa. There she received the intensive purification treatments known as Maharishi Rejuvenation therapy. Immediately after these treatments, she noticed that certain problems diminished.

Carrie continues to practice the Transcendental Meditation technique twice a day and has returned to The Raj for several rejuvenation treatments. She also follows her doctor's home care recommendations, including a diet to balance her doshas, Maharishi Yoga postures (asanas) and breathing exercises, Maharishi Ayur-Veda herbal supplements, and a natural, daily routine that includes Ayurvedic self-massage.

As a result of these treatments, Carrie has been able to stop taking most of her medications, except during mold season when she still occasionally needs Western drugs. She no longer has to take the drug that caused heart palpitations, and expects that her need for all drugs will eventually disappear altogether.

"I think the entire approach of Maharishi Vedic Medicine works really well," said Carrie. "It's the whole way of life that works. Maybe if you do just one of the approaches you'll get some relief, but if you do them all it's extremely powerful. That's what makes it different from other treatments."

Carrie notices many side benefits from her treatments. Painful neck and shoulder tension that used to wake her up at night disappeared. She lost excessive weight, and she no longer suffers from constipation. Practicing the Transcendental Meditation technique improved her mental focus and helped her artistic expression.

"I used to think, 'There will never be an end to this suffering. I'll have to do this the rest of my life,'" said Carrie. "But now I am beginning to feel well. Other people notice the change without knowing what I am doing. They say, 'Oh, you seem much calmer.'"

CHAPTER 12

Early Diagnosis: The Key to Effective Prevention and Treatment

"All influences on health—including physical, mental, and seasonal factors—are reflected in the pulse. Through the simple procedure of self-pulse reading, one can detect imbalances developing in the physiology in order to prevent disease through timely adjustment of diet and behavior. Self-pulse reading itself contributes some influence to the restoration of balance in the physiology. To achieve a disease-free society, it is necessary for all people to learn to read their own pulse."   —*Maharishi Mahesh Yogi*[32]

Many times, when patients seek the help of their doctors, they don't have any overt symptoms of disease but simply complain of vague feelings of discomfort. These patients may be bothered by inertia and lack of energy, for example, by a general feeling of discomfort and lack of well-being, or by nonspecific aches and pains. These individuals constitute a large portion of the patient population in Western countries. Physicians sometimes refer to them as the "worried well," an expression that indicates the prevailing attitude toward this group of patients. They are essentially healthy, they just worry too much. Allopathic medicine has little to offer such people, as their problems will not show up as physiological disorders in any diagnostic tests. The only thing allopathic physicians can do for such people is to send them home with the advice to get more rest. Alternatively, if the physician views such complaints as "all in the head," he or she may prescribe tranquilizers or antidepressants.

Maharishi Vedic Medicine considers this inability to read signals of disorder as clear disease symptoms to be one of the greatest limitations of allopathic medicine. Subtle feelings of discomfort or unease are important indicators of preclinical disorders, and ignoring them—or making matters worse by suppressing them with drugs—places the patient at great peril. Chronic disease develops insidiously over many years as physiological imbalances accumulate in the body. The patient's general feeling of malaise provides the only early warning signs that this is happening. At this stage, the disease process is still in its early stages, and the problem can be fairly easily corrected. By the time symptoms ppear, however, the imbalances are so deeply embedded in the mind-body system that they are considerably more difficult to eradicate.

Allopathic practitioners have little knowledge of the nature of mind-body imbalances, and they have no way to diagnose a problem if no observable symptoms are present. The patient has a vague sense that something is wrong, but cannot pinpoint its source. In contrast, Maharishi Vedic Medicine offers a number of sophisticated and subtle diagnostic techniques that allow the physician to detect imbalances long before they appear as symptoms.

Pulse Diagnosis

One of the most effective diagnostic tools available to the physician trained in Maharishi Vedic Medicine is called *nadi vigyan,* or pulse diagnosis. This traditional technique involves taking the patient's pulse to detect imbalances. Unlike allopathic practice, however, the doctor is not concerned with the beats per minute.

Rather, he or she places three fingers on the radial artery on the patient's wrist. Through this simple procedure, a trained physician can detect the state of balance or imbalance in the three doshas, the fifteen subdoshas, and the seven dhatus. The qualities of the doshas and the amount of ojas are also assessed. Based on this examination, the physician can prescribe therapies to address the subtle imbalances he or she detected.

Pulse diagnosis is a simple and straightforward technique, yet it is so powerful and accurate that it may seem almost like magic to

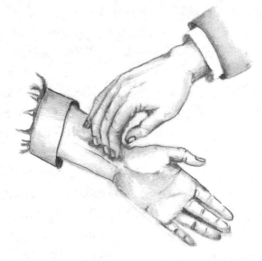

people who don't understand its mechanics. One of the most famous practitioners of nadi vigyan is the eminent Indian physician Dr. Brihaspati Dev Triguna. He is the private physician of the President of India and also runs a tremendously busy clinic in Delhi that offers free treatments for the poor. On a visit to the United States, Dr. Triguna was once asked to take the pulse of a skeptical newspaper reporter. He put his fingers on the reporter's pulse for only a moment. To the reporter's amazement, Dr. Triguna correctly noted that the reporter was color-blind and had recently passed a kidney stone.

Pulse diagnosis is an important tool both for preventing chronic disease and for diagnosing the cause of illness once symptoms have emerged. Many patients display not one, but many different symptoms. In such cases, it is important to identify the deepest source of imbalance. Once the primary imbalance is eliminated, the other disease manifestations often diminish automatically.

Rhonda, a housewife and mother, experienced first-hand the benefits of pulse diagnosis when she sought help for the extreme mood swings and fatigue she was experiencing before each menstrual period. Her primary physician had been unable to help her. Nothing showed up in the tests he ran, and his only suggestion had been to put her on antidepressants and tranquilizers, which Rhonda refused because she felt happy and normal most of the time.

Instead she decided to visit a Maharishi Vedic Medical Center. The physician took her pulse and told her that her problems were caused by an imbalance in two of her subdoshas, Ranjaka Pitta and Apana Vata. Ranjaka Pitta is involved in blood formation and Apana Vata governs elimination and the downward flow of menstruation. Irregular elimination had caused toxins to accumulate in her system, which in turn had thrown her hormones and other systems out of balance. By changing her diet and taking herbal food supplements to decrease Ranjaka Pitta and to improve elimination, Rhonda was able to reduce her mood swings drastically within a short period of time.

"It was a relief to have someone finally acknowledge that I had an actual problem," said Rhonda. "The physician accurately described my symptoms and their causes—without any verbal information from me. That gave me tremendous confidence in the pulse-diagnosis process. I felt I had finally found someone who really knew what was wrong with me and could do something about it."

Pulse diagnosis has another important benefit. It enables the physician to discriminate among different causes of disease, even for the same disorder. Bronchial asthma, for example, is considered one disease, yet it may originate from very different imbalances. For this reason, not everyone with the same disorder receives the same treatment. Treating all types of asthma in the same way would give unsatisfactory results and could even worsen the problem. The treatment programs in Maharishi Vedic Medicine are highly individualized. Each one is designed on the basis of the unique features of the individual patient's nervous system.

Self-Pulse Diagnosis

Self-pulse diagnosis is one of the most useful preventive techniques you can adopt to take control of your health. It enables you to read the subtle messages of your own pulse, helping you to stay in tune with the daily and seasonal fluctuations of the doshas and to detect imbalances so that you can address them before they take root. In addition, the very process of sensing the impulses of the pulse creates a balancing influence in the body. In taking the pulse, you bring the power of awareness, or consciousness, to the body.

Mothers can also learn to take the pulses of their children to keep them in perfect health. If a mother reads her child's pulse and finds an imbalance, she can simply adjust the child's diet or daily routine. The health of the entire family can be maintained in this way.

With the right instruction, self-pulse diagnosis is fairly simple to learn, but it's not a skill that can be picked up from a book. You must have an experienced teacher. Maharishi Vedic Universities throughout the United States offer courses in self-pulse diagnosis. To find out more about these courses, see the Appendix.

Other Diagnostic Tools

A physician trained in Maharishi Vedic Medicine uses many other tools to diagnose a disease. He or she will look at your individual and family medical history and in addition will consider a number of mental, physical and emotional characteristics. These include skin, hair and eye color, body build, digestive strength, regularity of elimination and urination, food preferences, mental qualities, lifestyle and behavioral tendencies, and emotional characteristics. The physician's questionnaire may include questions on how often you get angry or how much you worry, as well as more standard questions about your age and weight. Mental, emotional, and behavioral characteristics are given as much importance as physical attributes.

All of these qualities help the doctor assess your basic doshic makeup and your specific doshic imbalances. Remember that although all three doshas are always present in your physiology, their proportions vary in each individual. Almost everyone is born with a predominance of one or two doshas, but over a lifetime, deeply rooted patterns of behavior and habits can influence this basic doshic composition to such a degree that it appears to have changed. This altered doshic composition is referred to as your *deha prakriti*, or your current doshic constitution. Your Ayurvedic examination usually determines the deha prakriti. The physician takes the deha prakriti into account in determining the causes of disease, because it gives a clue to your strengths and weaknesses and tendencies for illness.

Apart from changes in the underlying doshic makeup, wrong dietary habits or unhealthy lifestyle patterns can create a state of imbalance in the doshas. This is called *vikriti*. For example, if your constitution is dominated by Vata but you eat lots of spicy foods, you may develop a Pitta imbalance—a Pitta vikriti—and experience Pitta-related disorders. Determining the exact nature of your vikriti is an important diagnostic step because it gives the physician important clues about how to restore the balance of the doshas before disease develops. The physician will also look at the strength and health of the tissues (dhatus), the compactness of the organs, the power of digestion, the quality of the mind, and the capacity for exercise. These factors help determine whether the treatment should be strong, moderate or mild.[33]

If the disease is complicated or advanced, small or has spread throughout the body, or has manifested as several diseases, the doshas are so out of balance that it may be hard to determine the primary source of illness through pulse diagnosis alone. Then the patient's history, habits, and lifestyle provide important indicators. Naturally, it is also to the patient's and doctor's advantage to use modern diagnostic tools as well, when they are useful. Maharishi Vedic Medicine is an important complement to conventional medicine, not a substitute for it. Sometimes both systems of medicine can ensure the best results.

Taking all these diagnostic factors into account, the physician can determine the ideal health care program targeted for the unique conditions of each individual's nervous system. The treatment program is never disease-specific. That is, it is never assigned to you just because you have a certain sickness. It is always prescribed on the basis of the specific conditions in your physiology that are causing that disorder.

Redefining the Doctor-Patient Relationship

People often feel isolated and estranged by the modern medical system. Allopathic physicians spend years in medical school learning about the many forms and expressions of disease. Is it any wonder that some get trapped into treating diseases rather than people? Dr. Eric Cassell wrote eloquently about this problem in his insightful book, *The Healer's Art: A New Approach to the Doctor-Patient Relationship.* "Scientific medicine deals with disease; its view of the world of the sick is the view of disease," he writes. "The manner in which physicians are trained quite naturally emphasizes and reinforces the current definitions of disease and the view of illness that such definitions promote. . . . Analytic thinking, which is so useful to physicians in understanding the body, leads away from considerations of the whole person and is in conflict with that within the doctor which would be more useful for his healing function."[34]

Many people using Maharishi Vedic Medicine report that it provides a qualitatively different experience. Rhonda felt reassured and comforted when she first started seeing a physician at a Maharishi Vedic Medical Center. Up until then, her primary care physician downplayed her discomfort, because none of the tests he ran showed evidence of any specific physiological disorders. Her Ayurvedic physician dealt with her problems as something concrete and real. For the first time she felt assured that she could talk about what she sensed her body was trying to tell her.

"I felt like I was being treated as a whole person. I wasn't just identified in terms of my disease," recalled Rhonda. "The physician took my complaints seriously and was able to immediately pick up on the problems I was experiencing. He took everything into account—my digestion, my emotional state and my thinking process. It was obvious that he was focusing on treating my whole physiology, and not just an isolated problem."

It was cases like Rhonda's that made me realize that dramatic changes were taking place in my own practice as a result of adding the knowledge of Maharishi Vedic Medicine to my allopathic training. I used to see isolated symptoms when I diagnosed. Now I see an aware, unique human being who has somehow stepped off the path of perfect health, but who has every possibility of becoming whole and healthy again. I can now convey hope and enthusiasm to my patients, because I have seen time and again how treatments can work with the subtle intelligence of the body—instead of against it—and help solve the problems of chronic disease. The therapies of Maharishi Vedic Medicine provide a simple, yet surprisingly effective, means of enlivening this powerful force of healing in the body. In the following chapters, you will learn about the many therapies through which disease can be transformed into health.

CHAPTER 13

Reconnecting with Consciousness

"Perfect health is wholeness. In its full meaning wholeness takes in everything: not only the body, but also the
mind, the environment and their past and future
continuity in time. It includes the society, the ecology,
and the universe in the outer extreme, and the abstract eternal realm of ideas and truth at the inner
level. Perfect health, or absolute wholeness, therefore
includes all these realms of life in a state of perfect
dynamic balance in a flow of optimum evolution."
—*Maharishi Mahesh Yogi*[35]

Everyone who knew Jerry thought he had a warm heart. He
and his wife, Mary, took loving care of their family of seven—including four foster children who suffered from multiple problems of mental retardation, autism, Alzheimer's and deafness.
However, the caliber of his emotions bore no relation to the condition of his physical heart. When he was only twenty-nine, he was
shocked to discover that he suffered from cardiomyopathy, a disease of the heart muscles.

"They said I only had six months or a year to live," he said.
Needless to say, he felt depressed and worried about the fate of
his family. None of the doctors he consulted offered any hope of
stopping the slow deterioration of his heart.

That was six years ago. Jerry started the Transcendental Meditation program soon after his diagnosis. He also started an Ayurvedic

diet, to perform Maharishi Yoga exercises, and to take a rejuvenating food supplement called Maharishi Amrit Kalash™. Jerry noticed his condition slowly improving. His cardiologists noticed too. Each year the echocardiogram indicated more healing in his heart. "About two or three years ago," he said, "the test showed my heart was perfectly normal."

Today Jerry can climb stairs on his exercise machine for over an hour—a big change from six years ago, when he had to stop and rest periodically. "None of the cardiologists know of any case where cardiomyopathy has ever reversed itself," he says. "But today my heart is completely healthy."

Although all the therapies of Maharishi Vedic Medicine work together, the development of consciousness is the cornerstone of the treatments. Like Jerry, millions of people have found that the Transcendental Meditation program can help them overcome debilitating problems and rejuvenate their minds and bodies beyond their expectations.

Violation of Natural Law is the basic cause of sickness. Wrong diet, detrimental lifestyle choices, and overexposure to stress all fall into this category. Of course, people generally don't violate Natural Law on purpose. Usually it is due to lack of knowledge—lack of understanding of what your body needs to stay healthy. All aspects of Maharishi Vedic Medicine make this information available—knowledge about proper diet, daily routine, seasonal routine, and so forth. However, practicing the TM technique is by far the most effortless way to produce a state of consciousness in which you start making spontaneous choices to promote health and stop making mistakes that damage it.

The TM program is the foundation of Maharishi Vedic Medicine's health care programs, because it connects individual awareness with its basis in pure consciousness, the total potential of Natural Law. When every thought and behavior is a simple, automatic expression of Nature's pure intelligence, violations of Natural Law, the root cause of sickness and suffering, cease to exist.

How the *Transcendental Meditation* Technique Improves Health

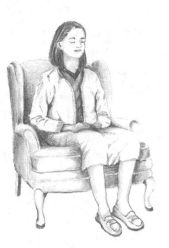

The TM program is a simple, effortless technique that provides extremely deep rest and eliminates stress from the mind and body. Simultaneously it opens the mind to its source, an infinite reservoir of energy, intelligence, creativity, organizing power, and bliss. The TM technique has been found to increase intelligence and improve emotional and physical health. It even creates a harmonious influence in society and the environment when enough people practice it. It takes only fifteen or twenty minutes twice a day, and is done while sitting with eyes closed in a comfortable chair. Commuters often practice it on the bus or train.

Anyone can learn the Transcendental Meditation technique, irrespective of age (from ten to 110 years), stress level, or educational or cultural background. People of all ages and from all walks of life notice benefits—from increased energy, productivity and motivation to enhanced mental clarity and creativity, from better health and well-being to improved performance in school and on the job. The elderly also benefit, because the deep rest rejuvenates and restores the mind-body, eliminating disease and slowing or reversing the aging process.

How to Learn

The Transcendental Meditation program requires personal instruction to be learned properly. A book cannot adequately convey how to do it. However, hundreds of Transcendental Meditation program centers and Maharishi Vedic Universities exist throughout the world where you can learn to meditate from a specially trained teacher. The course consists of seven steps, including two introductory lectures that you can attend free of charge. The third step is a brief personal interview. The fourth step provides personal instruction in the practice, and takes about an hour and a half. After that you attend three follow-up meetings on consecutive days—steps five, six, and seven—in which you receive more detailed instruction as well as a vision of the long-term, cumulative benefits of this meditation. The TM technique is so easy to learn that most students experience some benefits even in the first few days of practice. (See the Appendix to locate a teacher in your area.)

A Fourth State of Consciousness

One of the reasons that the TM technique is so helpful in the treatment of chronic disease is that it allows patients to experience a deeply restful fourth state of consciousness. You are probably already familiar with three states of consciousness—waking, sleeping, and dreaming. These are defined as distinct states of consciousness because the mind and body exhibit discrete, predictable modes of functioning with measurable parameters such as breath rate, metabolic rate, heart rate, and brainwave pattern.

Researchers have found that during the Transcendental Meditation technique, the body experiences a profound level of rest, indicated by such phenomena as decreased heart and breath rates and brief periods of suspended breathing. At the same time, the mind settles down effortlessly to its fundamental reservoir of inner silence or pure consciousness, where it is absolutely calm, yet fully awake. This produces a distinct brainwave pattern marked by high levels of coherence across specific frequencies. This unique state of mind and body, called "restful alertness," is a fourth major state of consciousness, which has its own predictable qualities.

This state of restful alertness yields many rewards. As a physician,

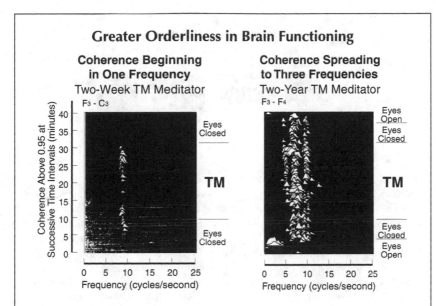

Greater Orderliness in Brain Functioning

Coherence Beginning in One Frequency
Two-Week TM Meditator

Coherence Spreading to Three Frequencies
Two-Year TM Meditator

Greater brain-wave coherence, along with the many other physiological changes produced by the Transcendental Meditation technique, suggests a unique style of neurophysiological functioning during the practice–a state of restful alertness. EEG coherence has been found to be correlated with higher levels of creativity, intelligence, moral reasoning, and neuromuscular efficiency, and with experiences of higher states of consciousness.

References: 1. P. Levine, "The Coherence Spectral Array (COSPAR) and its Application to the Study of Spatial Ordering on the EEG," *Proceedings of the San Deigo Biomedical Symposium* 15 (1976).
2. K. Badawi, R. K. Wallace, D. W. Orme-Johnson, and A. M. Rouzere, "Electrophysiologic Characteristics of Respiratory Suspension Periods Occurring During the Practice of the Transcendental Meditation Program, " *Psychosomatic Medicine* 46 (1984): 267-276.
3. D. W. Orme-Johnson, G. Clements, C. T. Haynes, and K. Badawi, "Higher States of Consciousness: EEG Coherence, Creativity, and Experiences of the Sidhis," in *Scientific Research on the* Transcendental Meditation *Program, Collected Papers, Volume 1,* ed. D. W. Orme-Johnson and J.T. Farrow (Livingston Manor, NY: MERU Press, 1977), 705-712.
4. M. C. Dillbeck and E. C. Bronson, "Short-Term Longitudinal Effects of the Transcendental Meditation Technique on EEG Power and Coherence," *International Journal of Neuroscience* 14 (1981): 147-157.

I see many patients who suffer from fatigue, stress, and anxiety. The Transcendental Meditation technique allows people to alleviate both cumulative and daily stress, to sleep deeply and think clearly, to decrease anxiety and increase energy and enthusiasm, and to experience happiness and well-being—to name just a few of

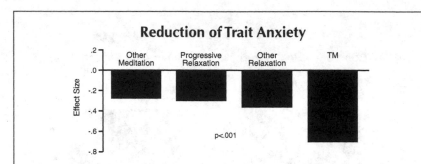

Reduction of Trait Anxiety

A statistical meta-analysis of all available studies (99 independent outcomes), indicated that the effect of the Transcendental Meditation program on reducing trait anxiety was approximately twice as great as that of all other meditation and relaxation techniques, including progressive muscle relaxation. Duration of the study, dropout rate, and number of follow-up hours of instructions were statistically controlled, and samples were matched for type of population. Analysis also showed that the positive result for the TM program could not be attributed to subject expectation, experimenter bias or quality of research design. Meta-analysis is the preferred scientific procedure for drawing definitive conclusions from large bodies of research.

The TM program produces a markedly greater reduction in general level of anxiety compared to relaxation procedures or other forms of meditation. This finding corroborates studies indicating that the TM technique produces substantially greater physiological effects than ordinary relaxation both during the practice and enduring over time. Research suggests that the highly distinctive state of restful alertness experienced during the TM technique neutralizes deep-rooted stresses in the nervous system, resulting in a wide range of physiological and psychological changes, such as reduced anxiety, improved physical health, and more rewarding behavior. A reduction in anxiety is typically accompanied by wide-ranging benefits in many areas of life.

References: 1. K. Eppley, A. Abrams, and J. Shear, "Differential Effects of Relaxation Techniques on Trait Anxiety: A Meta-analysis," *Journal of Clinical Psychology*, vol. 45 (1989), pp. 957-974.
2. Michael C. Dillbeck, "The Effect of the *Transcendental Meditation* Technique on Anxiety Level," *Journal of Clinical Psychology*, vol. 33 (1977), pp. 1076-1078.

the benefits. All of these results are vital for preventing and curing chronic disease. In short, it is just what the doctor ordered.

How the *Transcendental Meditation* Program
Helps Treat Chronic Disease

My patients who practice the Transcendental Meditation technique are often able to overcome the debilitating fear and anger that can accompany chronic disease. Patients frequently become sicker just from hearing a doctor tell them how ill they are. Many people lose hope, and some even become frantic.

The Transcendental Meditation technique does not simply help people manage emotional and physical stress, it reduces stress. In addition, practitioners find an ocean of inner silence and peace within themselves. When tension and anxiety levels decrease, and individuals develop a deeper sense of themselves, they stop feeling overwhelmed by pain and discomfort. Most importantly, the experience of restful alertness returns the mind and body to a state of equilibrium. This triggers the innate mechanisms that allow the body to heal itself. So many times I have seen that after only a few weeks of this practice, my patients feel renewed vitality and are able to take the necessary steps to recover from even the most debilitating diseases. The TM technique also helps in a number of other ways.

Eliminating the Cause of Disease

The primary source of disease is the disconnection of the infinite field of pure intelligence within us from our true nature. This same intelligence that creates and organizes the entire mind-body system also orchestrates the whole universe. The TM technique opens awareness to its unbounded source, this field of pure intelligence, on a daily basis, re-enlivening the connection between individual and universal consciousness. When access to, and eventually identity with, pure consciousness is restored, the mind-body is once again governed by the perfect managing intelligence of Nature. Obstructions to the flow of consciousness in the body are removed. The body's internal healing systems are rejuvenated and physiological balance is reestablished. The cause of present and future disease is thus eliminated.

Reducing Psychosomatic Illness

You probably have heard that at least 80 per cent of diseases are thought to be psychosomatic, that is, originating in the mind as well as the body. The Transcendental Meditation technique brings balance to the entire mind-body system and dramatically reduces mental, emotional, and physical stress, each of which can

---

Reduced Cardiovascular Risk Factor

Research published in American Heart Association journals *Stroke* and *Hypertension* shows that the Transcendental Meditation program:

• Significantly reduces blockage of blood vessels supplying blood to the brain and the heart without change in diet or exercise. These results correlated with a 11% reduction in risk of heart attack due to atherosclerosis, and a 7.7–15% reduction in risk of stroke due to atherosclerosis.

• Is twice as effective as other relaxation techniques in reducing hypertension without change in diet or exercise. These results correlated with a 35–40% reduction in risk of stroke due to hypertension and a 20–45% reduction in risk of coronary heart disease due to hypertension.

• Produces a 15% reduction in lipid peroxide (cholesterol) levels, associated with reduced risk for atherosclerosis.

References: 1. A. Castillo-Richmond, M.D. et al., "Effects of Stress Reduction on Cartoid Atherosclerosis in Hypertensive African Americans," *Stroke*, vol. 31 (2000), pp. 568–573.
2. R.H. Schneider, M.D. et al., "A Randomized Controlled Trial of Stress Reduction for Hypertension in Older African Americans," *Hypertension*, vol. 26 (1995), pp. 820–827.
3. C.N. Alexander et al., "A Trial of Stress Reduction for Hypertension in Older African Americans (Part II): Gender and Risk Subgroup Analysis," *Hypertension*, vol. 28 (1996), pp. 228–237.
4. R.H. Schneider, M.D. et al., "Lower Lipid Peroxide Levels in Practitioners of the *Transcendental Meditation* Program," *Psychosomatic Medicine*, vol. 60 (1998), pp. 38–41.

---

be a major factor in psychological distortion. Consequently, it is an extremely effective tool in combating psychosomatic diseases. Cardiovascular disease, bronchial asthma, mental illness, and digestive tract disorders are just a few of the psychosomatic diseases that have been shown by scientific research to improve with the use of the TM technique.

Reducing the Major Stress Factors

We live in a highly stressful world that creates a steady barrage

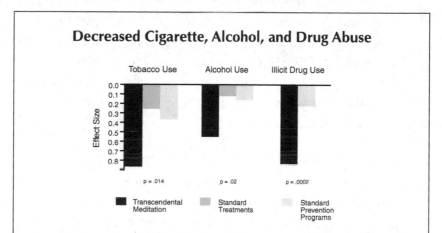

Decreased Cigarette, Alcohol, and Drug Abuse

A statistical meta-analysis of 198 independent treatment outcomes found that the Transcendental Meditation program produced a significantly larger reduction in tobacco, alcohol, and illicit drug use than either standard substance abuse treatments (including counseling, pharmacological treatments, relaxation training, and Twelve-step programs) or prevention programs (such as programs to counteract peer-pressure and promote personal development). This meta-analysis controlled for strength of study design and included both heavy and casual users. Whereas the effects of conventional programs typically decrease sharply by 3 months, effects of Transcendental Meditation on total abstinence from tobacco, alcohol, and illicit drug ranged from 51%-89% over an extended time.

Reference: 1. "Treating and preventing alcohol, nicotine, and drug abuse through Transcendental Meditation: A review and statistical meta-analysis," *Alcoholism Treatment Quarterly*, vol. 11 (1994), pp. 13–87
2. "Effectiveness of the Transcendental Meditation program in preventing and treating substance misuse: A review," *International Journal of the Addictions* No. 26 (1991). pp. 293–325.

of strong stimuli. Millions of Americans today complain of lifestyles so hectic that they don't have enough time to sleep or eat properly. Such demanding lifestyles constantly strain the mind and body. Unfortunately, many people resort to behaviors to escape stress that ultimately produce more stress and even disease. Alcohol and cigarettes, for example, bring some kind of relaxation and relief from mental tension, but they also take a deadly toll on the body.

When my patients begin the Transcendental Meditation program, they immediately start to feel more relaxed. Spontaneously, they stop desiring damaging substances such as cigarettes, alcohol, drugs, and even caffeine. As energy and inner happiness grow, they see artificial mood- and energy-boosters as blocks to their body's functioning, which is actually the case. They become more in tune with their minds and bodies, with Nature itself, and begin to make better choices. All of this adds up to a lifestyle that supports health.

On the radio the other day, I heard a leading cardiologist commenting on new advertisements that are meant to frighten smokers into quitting. The cardiologist said flatly that the advertisements are useless. "The problem is not motivating people to quit smoking," he said. "The problem is teaching people how to quit." In other words, even if a person wants to quit, he or she may not be able to do so. Research shows that the Transcendental Meditation program is highly effective in helping people to break addictive habits—including smoking—that lead to disease.

The *TM-Sidhi* Program and Collective Health

Although we have focused mainly on the Transcendental Meditation technique in this chapter, Maharishi Vedic Medicine includes many other technologies to develop higher states of consciousness. One such technique is the TM-Sidhi program, which can be learned after a person has been practicing the TM tech-

Chronic Diseases Helped by the
***Transcendental Meditation* Technique**

Disorder	Per cent Improvement
Cardiovascular	92
Digestive tract	69
Musculoskeletal	94
Nose, throat, lung	89
Neurological	76
Glandular and metabolic	93
Mental health and substance abuse	92
Infectious disease	93
Skin disorder	86
Blood disorder	41

Reference: David W. Orme-Johnson, Ph D, and Robert E. Hernon, Ph D, "An Innovative Approach to Reducing Medical Care Utilization and Expenditures", *American Journal of Managed Care*, 1997, 3:135–144

nique regularly for a few months. While the TM technique opens the individual mind to the underlying field of pure consciousness, the TM-Sidhi program cultures the ability to think and act from this level, strongly enhancing mind-body coordination and producing gradual mastery over the Laws of Nature. Practitioners learn to think and act from the deepest level of Natural Law from where the entire universe is created and maintained.

The TM-Sidhi program enlivens certain Laws of Nature that are expressed in the human system as specific areas of functioning. Some, for example, refine emotions while others enhance sensory perception. Through the practice, each area of the nervous system involved in these functions is purified, while mind-body coordination is strengthened. The "master" technique in the TM-Sidhi program is "Yogic Flying," which develops the ability to move through the air by virtue of a thought or simple intention—

a clear display of unobstructed mind-body coordination. During the first stage of Yogic Flying, the body lifts up and moves forward in short hops. The experience is one of exhilaration, lightness, and joy, as individual awareness must be grounded in the blissful field of pure consciousness in order to lift off successfully.

Research verifies that brain wave activity becomes completely coherent at the time the body lifts up. Consequently, people who practice Yogic Flying experience increased ability to think clearly and creatively and to accomplish both immediate and long-term goals effectively. The TM-Sidhi program cultivates a high degree of neurophysiological refinement throughout the mind-body, resulting in better health, psychophysiological stability and balance, decreased stress, more happiness, and more support from the environment.

This is interesting from the perspective of conquering chronic disease, because as the mind becomes more in tune with the managing

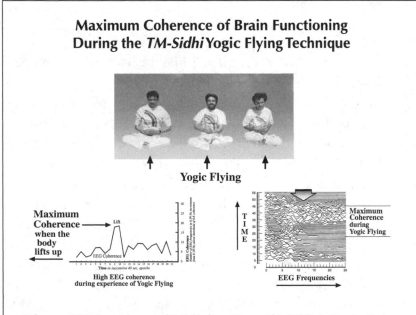

Maximum Coherence of Brain Functioning During the *TM-Sidhi* Yogic Flying Technique

Yogic Flying

Maximum Coherence when the body lifts up

High EEG coherence during experience of Yogic Flying

Maximum Coherence during Yogic Flying

EEG Frequencies

Reference: D.W. Orme-Johnson and P. Gelderloos, "Typographic EEG Brain Mapping During Yogic Flying," *International Journal of Neuroscience.*

intelligence of Nature, it spontaneously makes healthier choices that prevent disease. However, Yogic Flying is significant for another reason as well. It has a dramatic impact on collective health.

The scope of Maharishi Vedic Medicine includes not only individual health, but also the health of society. Group practice of the Transcendental Meditation and TM-Sidhi programs creates a powerful influence of coherence and peace in the environment, reducing collective stress and its symptoms, such as crime and sickness. More than thirty studies show that group practice of Yogic Flying can lower a community's crime and accident rates, hospital admissions, and even incidents of war-related violence. One dramatic example of this type of intervention took place in 1993, when 4,000 Yogic Flyers from around the world traveled to Washington, D.C., to practice the Transcendental Meditation and TM-Sidhi programs together. During the four-week demonstration period, Washington's crime rate dropped significantly, and this drop could not be explained by any other interventions.

How can practicing a technique to develop individual potential affect the whole society? The field of consciousness provides a lively yet invisible connection among all peoples and between human life and the entire universe. Every aspect of creation is an expression of consciousness. When an imbalance arises in individual life, it affects society, or collective consciousness, as well. When even a small pebble falls in a pond, it creates ripples that spread through the water. Similarly, every impulse of every individual awareness stirs the ocean of consciousness shared by all. When enough people radiate stress and unhappiness, the ripples can become turbulent waves and indicators of collective negativity such as war, crime, family violence, epidemics, and economic failure. When society is sufficiently imbalanced, it is vulnerable to sickness.

Fortunately, it is easier to dissolve this collective stress than you may think. Research has shown that even a small number of individuals—approximately the square root of one per cent of the population—practicing the Transcendental Meditation and TM-Sidhi programs together generate a sufficiently powerful influence of orderliness, harmony, and health to reestablish balance in the collective mind-body. This has come to be known as the Maharishi Effect.

The group practice of meditation was an integral part of Ayur-Veda at its inception. The Ayurvedic texts recount that the eternal knowledge of Ayur-Veda was imparted to the great *rishi* (seer) Bharadwaja during a meeting of all the enlightened sages. Even though healthy themselves, the wise men assembled because they were concerned that disease had begun to afflict mankind. In the deep silence and coherence created by their collective meditation, Ayur-Veda, "the knowledge of life," was understood by Bharadwaja.[37]

Growing up in India, I often heard the expression *Vasudhaiva kutumbakam*—"the world is my family." It is comforting to me as a physician, a mother, and a member of the world family to know that the collective health of the whole world can be attended to by this branch of Maharishi Vedic Medicine. Surely no one who feels any amount of compassion can be completely happy and fulfilled if others are suffering. Surely no one in this day of the "global village" can feel that health is just an individual matter. We live in a time when the economic, political, and health trends in every corner of the world can directly affect every individual on the globe. Until we erase the possibility of war, famine and crime from our planet, none of us can be assured of perfect health for ourselves or our families.

CHAPTER 14

The Importance of Diet in Creating Balance and Healing

"Food sustains the life of living beings. All living beings in the universe require food. Complexion, clarity, good voice, longevity, genius, happiness, satisfaction, nourishment, strength, and intellect are all conditioned by food."
—Charaka Samhita[38]

Tony claims that he never touched a vegetable for the first twenty-two years of his life. He ate a diet rich in hot spices, meat, cheese, and other heavy foods. Despite the intense demands of his financial consulting business, he still managed to spend plenty of time soaking up the sun. He was born with a fair, delicate skin, yet his sun-worshiping habits had turned his skin a deep brown. What he didn't realize was that his deep tan, as well as the dry air and plentiful sunshine of Phoenix, Arizona masked severe psoriasis.

After moving to a small Midwestern town and braving the dry, cold winter there, Tony found his skin started to erupt. "No part of my body went untouched," Tony says of the psoriasis that ravaged his body. "What wasn't red and inflamed was white, flaky, and falling off." He couldn't sleep at night, couldn't focus at work, couldn't see other people. "I virtually had to drop out of society," Tony remembers.

Although the psoriasis emerged quite suddenly, Tony was very familiar with the disease. Most of his close family members suffered from it. They covered it cosmetically or treated it with steroids. "My family felt that psoriasis was untreatable, something you just have to manage," he said. "But I wasn't satisfied to spend the rest of my life like that. I wanted to find another way."

Through friends he heard about Maharishi Vedic Medicine. "At my first appointment, the doctor explained that my condition was caused by a Pitta imbalance and by toxins, or ama, that had accumulated in my body from years of eating foods that weren't suitable for my physiology," Tony recalls.

The doctor told Tony that although it might take a while, he felt confident that his condition would eventually disappear. He put Tony on a Pitta-pacifying diet and, to prevent additional ama formation, instructed him to minimize the intake of meat and other foods that were difficult to digest. To help unload the backlog of impurities that were at the root of Tony's psoriasis, he recommended that Tony undergo Maharishi Rejuvenation therapy as a seasonal purification treatment.

Tony diligently followed the recommendations, modifying his diet and receiving the purification treatments three times a year. "It was eat broccoli or die," he said with a laugh. He adhered faithfully to the Pitta-balancing regime, avoiding hot spices, cheese, onions, garlic, and other heat-producing foods. He stopped eating red meat and switched to chicken and fish. He eventually lost the desire for meat altogether. He also stayed out of the sun, because the doctor explained to him that sunlight increases Pitta, which would exacerbate his skin problems.

Since Tony's condition resulted from a lifelong indulgence in Pitta-aggravating and ama-producing foods and behaviors, it did not vanish overnight. However, as soon as he changed his diet, he felt an immediate improvement in his well-being. Eventually, his inflamed skin started to clear up and the red, itchy patches disappeared completely within a few weeks. "Once the condition started to turn, it went so quickly, it was fairly miraculous," recalls Tony. Today, at age thirty-seven, Tony enjoys a normal life without psoriasis, a disease that mainstream medicine considers incurable. To avoid a relapse, Tony is careful to live a balanced life. He avoids heat-producing foods and other influences that could aggravate Pitta or increase ama in his system.

As Tony's example illustrates, your daily diet affects your health in many important ways. Diet is one of the pillars of health in Maharishi Vedic Medicine. Eating is one of the three most significant things you do each day to renew your body and uphold health. The right foods can not only prevent disease, but also alleviate many chronic problems. Changing harmful dietary habits is one of the simplest, yet most effective, steps you can take to eliminate chronic disease. Conversely, foods that don't support your particular doshic constitution can lead to imbalances that eventually turn into disease. As the *Charaka Samhita* puts it, "A self-controlled man can live for one hundred years free from disease through the intake of wholesome food."[39]

It can be difficult to know what to eat and what not to eat. The popular press today tells you to eat oat bran to lower cholesterol, take antioxidant vitamins, and cook with the right vegetable oils. Tomorrow, however, these nutritional guidelines could change. A few years ago, experts told you to lower your cholesterol by eating unsaturated fats. Then researchers found that some unsaturated fats—such as the polyunsaturated fats in corn oil and safflower oil—can contribute to colon cancer. No wonder you get confused.

Even when the nutritional guidelines are generally helpful, they usually don't tell you anything about the importance of individual considerations. No one diet fits all people. One of the unique features of Maharishi Vedic Medicine is that it provides dietary guidelines tailored to each individual. Each person has different dietary needs, and even these change with seasonal factors and the state of personal health. Even two people suffering from the same disease may have significant variations in dietary needs. Though their symptoms are similar, their doshic makeup may differ and their illness could be caused by different imbalances.

Take the example of a person suffering from chronic head-aches. This condition can be caused by an imbalance in Vata or Pitta dosha. Determining the correct diet is even more difficult if the person is a heavy Kapha type, which could make him assume that he needs to eat light foods to lose weight. However, light foods increase Vata, which could further aggravate the underly-ing factors causing the chronic headaches.

To get a complete picture of the body's dietary needs, Maharishi Vedic Medicine uses pulse diagnosis and other diag-nostic measures to precisely assess the body's imbalances. The physician can then prescribe the most beneficial regime for each person. Maharishi Vedic Medicine uses diet to address chronic disease in several ways:

To purify body and mind

A heavy, sluggish pulse indicates that ama has lodged in the body and is obstructing the flow of the body's inner intelligence. In Chapter 7, you learned that ama is created by poor digestion. It is a sticky, heavy substance that can travel from the small intes-tine to any part of the body, blocking the srotas, or the circulatory channels, and sowing the seeds of future imbalances. Clogged ar-teries, cancer, and psoriasis are indications of severe ama accumu-lation, but the presence of ama can also show up as minor health problems and as general fatigue and tiredness. Diet can be used to reduce ama and prevent its production.

To correct imbalances

As you have seen, chronic disease involves severe and deep-rooted disturbances in the functioning of the doshas. Once the physician has determined which doshas are disturbed, he or she can give specific dietary recommendations to rebalance them. As simple as it may seem, individualized diet is one of the most potent and inexpensive ways of recreating health.

To nourish the dhatus and create ojas

Many people with chronic disease also become weak or malnourished because the srotas—the body's channels of transport that carry nutrient fluid—have been blocked by ama. A diet composed of nourishing, easily absorbed foods helps restore the health of the dhatus.

To prevent disease

Once disease is effectively treated, diet is one of the most efficient ways to keep the doshas balanced. If you eat food that is appropriate for your doshic constitution and make the dietary adjustments required by seasonal changes, you can maintain a healthy physiological equilibrium and prevent future imbalances.

The Ama-Reducing Diet

Increasing the power of agni is the key to eliminating ama. You may remember that strong agni can burn away existing pockets of ama and prevent new impurities from building up. When it isn't weighed down by digestive overload, the body's own self-regulating mechanisms automatically start to remove ama, eliminating impurities through the bowels, bladder and skin.

To understand how it is possible to reduce ama by changing what you eat, think of digestion as a kind of furnace. If you throw too much fuel on the fire, it gets snuffed out. Instead of a bright flame of heat, there is only smoke and ashes. This is what happens when people eat foods that are too heavy, eat at the wrong time, or eat before the previous meal has been digested. Digestion gets overwhelmed and food isn't processed properly. The outcome is often constipation, which further aggravates the problem by causing the unprocessed food to putrefy. This creates impurities that collect in the body and cause disease.

An ama-reducing diet kindles agni and strengthens digestion. It consists of foods that are nourishing, light, and easy to metabolize. Once the digestive powers are revived, heavier foods can be gradually added to the diet. It's just like starting a campfire: You start with kindling and add larger logs once the fire is going.

To start the fire, avoid foods that are difficult to digest and create ama, including meat, mushrooms, and packaged, processed, frozen, and canned foods. Many people love chocolate, but unfortunately it generates ama because it is difficult to digest and inhibits agni. The ideal diet is vegetarian, because it is light and easier to process, whereas meat is heavy and difficult to metabolize. Meat tends to produce ama and impurities in the colon, which then spread to other parts of the body. This is one of the reasons that vegetarians are known to have a lower incidence of heart disease, colon cancer, prostate cancer, and a number of other chronic or life-threatening diseases.

Additionally, eat organically grown foods as much as possible. Unfortunately pesticides, insecticides, and chemical fertilizers have been part of food production in our society for more than thirty years. They can lodge in the fat cells of the body, and these accumulated toxins generate many undesirable results. Some have hormone-like effects that can throw off the body's delicate hormonal balance. Others can trigger carcinogenic changes in the body. Some scientists hypothesize that the increase in breast cancer witnessed during the last thirty years is due to the buildup of toxins in the fatty breast tissue.

By purchasing organic foods, you escape the dangers of pesticides and insecticides altogether. This will also enable you to avoid eating foods that are genetically engineered. A number of scientists are alarmed at the widespread adoption of genetically altered foods in America, because the effects of these foods on the human body and the environment have not been adequately tested. At present, the organic label guarantees that the food is genetically unaltered.

Pure water is as important as pure food. It's worthwhile to get your water supply tested. If your drinking water has a high content of lead or pesticides, use bottled spring water instead, or install a water purifier in your home to remove foreign chemicals.

Rebalancing the Doshas

Diet is not only a therapeutic measure for reducing ama, it is

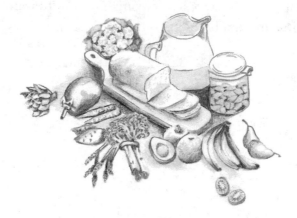

also one of the best ways to balance the doshas. Chapter 6 explained that Maharishi Vedic Medicine uses the principle of "like increases like" to determine the right diet to correct a doshic imbalance. According to this principle, the properties of the food you eat will increase the dosha with similar properties. If you have a strong Pitta imbalance, for example, you have too much heat in your system. Continuous consumption of foods with heating properties—for example, hot, spicy foods—further increases Pitta. If you continue eating heat-producing foods, you may eventually develop a Pitta-based disorder. If you change your diet, however, and start to eat foods with cooling properties—such as milk, wheat, or rice—the cooling properties will ease your aggravated Pitta and prevent further imbalances.

Maharishi Vedic Medicine does not classify foods according to their calories, fat content or food group. Instead, it emphasizes the six tastes of sweet, sour, salty, astringent, bitter and pungent. These six tastes have a profound effect on the doshas. Certain tastes increase certain doshas, while other tastes pacify them. For example, sweet tastes increase Kapha but decrease Vata and Pitta. A truly balanced meal includes all six tastes. Even if you eat to correct Kapha, using astringent, bitter, and pungent tastes, you still need to include some degree of the other three tastes in every meal to maintain physiological balance. The difference among the Vata, Pitta and Kapha diets is the *degree* to which each taste is favored.

The Six Tastes	
Taste	**Sample foods**
Sweet	Sugar, milk, butter, rice, breads, pasta
Sour	Yogurt, lemon, cheese
Salty	Salt and salty preparations
Pungent	Spicy foods, ginger, hot peppers, cumin
Bitter	Green leafy vegetables, bitter gourd, turmeric, fenugreek
Astringent	Beans, lentils, pomegranate, honey

When you have a consultation with a physician trained in Maharishi Vedic Medicine, you receive detailed dietary recommendations and a list of foods that will help nourish your body and eliminate the basis of disease. The diet uses the qualities of the six tastes and the principle of "like increases like" to address your specific doshic imbalances. There are three main diets, each of which aims at balancing one of the doshas. You need to consult with a physician to get a complete picture of your personal dietary needs, but here are a few major guidelines:

The Three Main Diets		
To Balance	**Favor**	**Minimize**
Vata	1. Warm, heavy and oily foods 2. Foods with sweet, sour and salty tastes 3. Eat larger quantities, but not more than you can digest easily	1. Cold, dry and light foods 2. Foods with pungent, bitter and astringent tastes.
Pitta	1. Foods that are liquid and cool in nature (but avoid ice-cold foods and drinks, as these inhibit digestion) 2. Foods with sweet, bitter or astringent tastes	1. Foods that are hot in temperature or properties 2. Foods with spicy, salty or sour tastes
Kapha	1. Light, dry and warm foods 2. Foods with pungent, bitter, and astringent tastes	1. Heavy, oily and cold foods 2. Foods with sweet, salty and sour tastes

Once your body has regained its doshic equilibrium and you no longer suffer from chronic disease, you can focus on preventing future illness by eating nourishing foods that maintain balance in the mind-body. You may need to rely more on prescribed dietary suggestions at first. Too many people are numb to their body's signals and are conditioned to eat unhealthy foods. Their body's natural intelligence has become clouded by imbalances and impurities which have built up over time. Once the body is free of these impurities and restored to its natural balance, however, you begin to feel more in tune with the body's needs and desires. You automatically become aware of the subtle signals that alert you to what's good for your body and what isn't. When you are in tune with your body's needs, you'll spontaneously eat the foods you need to maintain health.

Foods that Generate Ojas

Different foods create different influences in your body and mind. Some foods create lightness, softness and a feeling of peace. Others stimulate excitement or aggression, while others make you feel dull. Foods that are rich, fresh, and sweet are considered to be ideal because they enhance mental clarity as well as feelings of peace, purity and compassion. Three foods in particular create ojas and have a generally beneficial influence.

Milk

Milk has important nutritional properties, and is one of the best foods for balancing Pitta and Vata. A glass of warm milk at bedtime with a pinch of ginger nourishes the body and calms the mind. Maharishi Vedic Medicine recommends that you boil the milk, so that it creates less congestion and is easier to digest. This procedure is helpful even if you do not have trouble digesting milk.

You can also do a few other things to gain the most from this important food. Add two pinches of ginger, turmeric, or cardamom to the milk before boiling it. The spices aid digestion and help reduce Kapha. You can also add raw sugar or honey. (If honey, wait to add until the milk has cooled a bit.) Avoid drinking milk along with salty food or foods of mixed tastes, because this will make the milk hard to digest and create ama. It is better to drink milk at least one hour before or one hour after a meal to avoid mixing it with other foods. The only exception to this rule is if you're eating foods with sweet tastes, such as breakfast cereal, toast, rice, sugar or ghee.

Ghee (clarified butter)

The Ayurvedic texts ascribe numerous beneficial properties to ghee. Because of its many healing effects, it is one of the most important foods in treating chronic disease. Taken in moderation, ghee helps to balance all three doshas and improves digestion in several ways. For one, it enhances the flavor of food, increasing the appetite, kindling agni, and stimulating the secretion of digestive juices. Using ghee in foods promotes digestive power and facilitates assimilation.[40] By strengthening the digestive process, ghee boosts the output of ojas—the finest product of the digestive process. It also supports mental functioning, improving intelligence, memory, and understanding.

Ghee is one of the best fats for the body. It digests easily because it consists of short-chain fatty acids. Saturated animal and vegetable fats, on the other hand, are composed of long-chain fatty acids that are more difficult for the body to absorb. Ghee has an absorption rate of 96 per cent, the highest of all oils and fats. It does not increase cholesterol to the same extent as other fats. It has 8 per cent lower saturated fatty acids than butter, and the boiling process through which ghee is produced removes the protein casein, which has been linked to elevated cholesterol.

Ghee contains vitamins A, D, E, and K. Vitamins A and E are powerful antioxidants that play a key role in preventing damage from free radicals. Vitamin A also helps keep the outer lining of the eyeball moist, contributing to the health of the eye. In addition, ghee contains 4 to 5 per cent linoleic acid, an essential fatty acid that promotes the growth and renewal of the body. Many Ayurvedic medicines use ghee as a carrier because it facilitates the delivery of the medicinal properties to the tissues, increasing the effects of the herbs.

Making Ghee

To make ghee at home, simmer sweet (unsalted) butter until the foam and the milk solids sink to the bottom. This filters out water, fats and sugars.

When the solids have cooked and settled and the liquid is clear, the temperature of the ghee will rapidly increase, so at this point be alert to remove the ghee from the stove before it burns.

Place the pot on a cool surface, such as a pad or trivet, or in your sink. When it has cooled somewhat, pour the liquid ghee through cheesecloth or a fine-mesh strainer into a clean, dry jar.

Store the ghee at room temperature—not in the refrigerator. It will become a soft solid that will remain good for months.

You can also buy ghee through commercial outlets. For more information, see the "Resources" section in the Appendix.

Honey

Maharishi Vedic Medicine classifies honey as one of the seven most beneficial foods. It is an especially good sweetener for Kapha types, because it increases the digestive fire, opens the srotas, and helps rid the body of toxins. The valuable effects of honey are derived only from raw, unheated honey, however. Cooked honey or honey in baked foods in fact has an opposite effect on the srotas. It clogs these fine circulatory channels and blocks the flow of energy and intelligence in the body. Ayurvedic texts say that cooked honey is not only difficult to digest, but is even toxic. If you like honey in tea or warm milk, add the honey only after the liquid has cooled to a temperature that is comfortable for drinking.

General Dietary Principles for Avoiding Chronic Disease

Anyone with a chronic disease needs to consult a physician trained in Maharishi Vedic Medicine for an individualized diet based on doshic constitution and current imbalances. However, following certain general principles will help. The foods recommended here are light and easy to digest, and therefore increase agni, prevent ama production, and support balanced digestion.

In this chapter, you have seen the tremendous influence of diet on health. Through Maharishi Vedic Medicine, you can learn to eat the foods that awaken your body's healing ability, create balance, treat chronic disease and prevent future disease. The foods you eat are only half the story, however. The processes involved in transforming food into the body's building blocks are equally important. The therapeutic significance of digestion and the means for enhancing it will be the topic of the next chapter.

General Dietary Principles for Avoiding Chronic Disease

Avoid: Fried, oily food, leftover, packaged, cold foods. Heavy foods such as cheese, bananas, avocados, potatoes, and yogurt. *Lassi*, a drink made from *fresh* yogurt and water, is all right.

Spices that aid digestion: Cumin, cinnamon, fennel, cardamom, curry leaves

Helpful grains: Couscous, polenta, quinoa, barley in some cases, occasional *chapatis* (unleavened flat bread)

Vegetables: Favor asparagus, artichokes, zucchini, snow peas, fresh green beans
In lesser quantity: spinach, carrots, cabbage

Avoid: Broccoli and cauliflower

Fruit: Eat at room temperature, not cold. Favor pears, grapes, sweet fruit, sweet raspberries, apples

Avoid: Sour oranges and sour fruit

Other helpful foods:

Sweeteners: jaggary (a natural form of sugar available in Indian grocery stores)

Snacks: soaked almonds, raisins, figs

CHAPTER 15

Strengthening Digestion and Immunity

"Alleviation and aggravation of all the doshas are dependent upon the power of digestion and metabolism. Therefore, it is always necessary to maintain agni and avoid factors responsible for vitiating it."

—*Charaka Samhita*[41]

Food is one of the most important resources for creating health on a day-to-day basis. However, what you do with the food you eat is equally significant. Good digestion is the key to immunity, strength, and well-being. If your body can't properly process the food you eat, it doesn't matter how healthy your diet is. Without strong digestion, you won't derive the full nutritional value from food, and the waste products from weak digestion will further undermine your health. According to Maharishi Vedic Medicine, poor digestion and its destructive by-product—ama—is the key factor in the development of chronic disease. In general, if you see a person with chronic disease, you see a person who also suffers from chronic digestive problems.

Healthy digestion results from living in tune with your body and its inherent rhythms. Unfortunately, contemporary lifestyles violate the many subtle laws that regulate the body's digestive processes. Many people, for example, eat lightly at lunch when their digestive powers are strongest, then load up with a heavy evening meal even though the digestive fire is much weaker at night.

Many working professionals are too busy to take time to sit down and eat a meal. Instead they eat fast food on the run, while driving their cars or walking down the street. They frequently skip meals or eat at irregular times. Although such habits seem innocuous on the surface, they are highly detrimental to the finely tuned digestive process, which must be treated with care and attentiveness to function properly.

Weak digestion shows up in many ways—as feeling sluggish after meals, loss of appetite, constipation, loose stools, gas, headaches, and even mood swings. Your digestion affects your quality of life in more ways than you imagine. One of my patients, 33-year-old Rita, had suffered from low blood sugar, migraine headaches, dizziness, and menstrual problems for eleven years when she came to see me. She had been on an odyssey, traveling from medical doctors to chiropractors to acupuncturists, without any substantial improvement in her symptoms. An optometrist by profession, Rita finally learned about Maharishi Vedic Medicine from one of her patients.

When I took her pulse, it immediately became clear that Rita's problems had their source in weak digestion. Her situation was complicated by a diet that didn't support her doshic constitution or compensate for her poor digestive power. I explained how she should change her diet, eating habits, and lifestyle to alleviate these problems, and I also gave her some herbal supplements to normalize her digestion and balance the doshas more quickly.

That was all it took. "I don't quite understand how such simple measures could be so effective," Rita said, "but I've experienced what I would call a dramatic turnaround. In the eight months since I've begun treatments, I've only had one migraine headache. Before, I was getting them once a week, along with nausea, vomiting, and pain that kept me awake all night long. Also, now I can eat three meals without snacking all day, yet I don't have problems with low blood sugar attacks."

Digestive strength differs from person to person. Some people can consume large amounts of food while others eat less than half a plate. It is important to know your digestive capacity so you can avoid violating the delicate digestive process by eating too much. Digesting food is like cooking rice in a pot. For the rice to turn out perfectly, you need to have the right amount of water, of heat, and rice. If you turn the heat on too high, the rice will burn. If you turn the heat on too low, it will never get done. Too much agni, too little, or abnormal agni all cause problems in the body.

The Four Types of Agni

Samagni. This is normal or balanced agni. It digests food efficiently without producing excessive waste, burning, gas, or other digestive problems.

Vishmagni (erratic). This kind of agni fluctuates from meal to meal, and causes gas, pain in the abdomen, constipation, and other obstructions to normal elimination. It is often linked to Vata aggravation.

Tikshnagni (powerful or strong). This imbalance is associated with too much agni. In this case, even large amounts of food get digested too soon, producing burning in the abdomen, sour taste, thirst, heat in the body, and other problems. It is often created by excess Pitta.

Mandagni (weak, dull). Here the digestion is slow, and even small amounts of food take longer than normal to digest. Heaviness in the abdomen, dullness, and breathing trouble are some of the symptoms associated with this disorder. It develops from having too much Kapha and from eating between meals.

Digestive strength is assessed in part by how hungry you are before meals and how you feel after you eat. If your digestive fire is balanced, you will feel hungry before meals, digest all your food thoroughly, and feel light and clear after eating. If your digestive fire is irregular, too strong, or dull, you need to focus on improving your eating habits. Most health problems are caused by dull, weak digestion, where the food stays in the system for so long that you rarely feel hungry between meals.

The quality of digestion is often linked to the body's predominant dosha. An abundance of Vata tends to produce irregular digestion. Pitta dominance creates sharp, strong digestion. A prevalence of Kapha engenders mild or duller digestion. If you feel dull and heavy, you may have a Kapha-dominated agni. If you feel bloated or have gas, your agni may be Vata-dominant.

Your digestion, then, is affected both by the foods you eat and by your digestive efficiency. However, it is also influenced by how you prepare food and the conditions under which you eat it, such as fast food on the run versus lovingly prepared food in a settled environment.

Preparing Nourishing, Easily Digestible Foods

Eat fresh, unprocessed food

When you eat, you ingest the intelligence and the energy of Nature. Nutritional scientists long ago discovered that natural and freshly picked foods have a higher nutritional value. What scientists describe in terms of nutritional value can also be understood in terms of the degree to which Nature's intelligence is present in the food you eat. As long as the food is fresh and alive, the full value of intelligence and order is present. However, as the food ages, this value diminishes—the very process of aging involves a gradual breakdown of orderliness. If your diet is dominated by canned, frozen, or processed foods that sit on the supermarket shelves for months, you are impairing one of the most important mechanisms for upholding health on a day-to-day basis.

Old or processed foods are not only nutritionally diminished, but also harder to digest and therefore increase ama in the body. For the same reasons, try to avoid leftovers. Fresh vegetables and fruits, whole grains, and fresh breads are both nourishing and easy to digest. Once you start to use these types of food in your diet, you will notice an immediate improvement in your energy level and well-being.

Eat warm, well-cooked meals

Many people assume that raw foods are healthier because they have been processed less than cooked foods and therefore should retain more of their nutritional value. Raw foods are heavy to digest, however, and therefore often interfere with the digestive process. For this reason, the Ayurvedic texts emphasize that food should be well-cooked and eaten warm. Warm, deliciously cooked foods are more easily digested and soothe the digestive tract.

Raw foods are especially aggravating to Vata dosha because they are difficult to digest and create gas. However, a small amount of raw salad greens with grated beets, carrots, and fresh ginger can help stimulate your appetite at the beginning of a meal. People with more Kapha can benefit from eating a little more raw food to add lightness to their diet, but the main portion of the meal should consist of cooked food.

Prepare food with love

In Vedic times, the cook was revered for maintaining the health of the family for whom he cooked. If someone fell ill, the first questions asked were, "Is the cook happy? How was the food prepared?" In contemporary life, the art of cooking has been nearly forgotten, sacrificed to the innumerable demands on our time. Many people eat their meals out, living on food prepared by people who don't know them and who may even hate to cook.

The Ayurvedic texts state that the consciousness of the cook is transmitted to the food. Consequently, meals prepared by someone who loves you will have a very different effect from the food you buy from a stranger in a fast-food restaurant. When a loved one cooks for you with feelings of warmth and affection, nourishing qualities of love and friendship flow into the food. This has a powerful effect on how you feel and behave.

Make the food look and taste delicious

Every meal should look appetizing, taste delicious, and smell so good that you start salivating from the aroma alone. This will enhance your digestion and enable you to derive more nutritional value from the food than if the meal is bland and unappealing. You can make food more delicious by sautéing the vegetables in ghee with various spices and herbs. Spices add flavor, aid digestion, and, if used selectively, have a tremendous influence in balancing the doshas.

Eat with awareness, and involve all the five senses

Listen to the crunch of the vegetables and smell the aromas. Enjoy the shapes and colors and savor the different taste qualities of each item. You might even feel the textures of the food by eating with your hands. In most classical cultures, people eat with their hands, because touching adds life to the food.

Eating Habits That Improve Digestion

Do not overeat

According to Maharishi Vedic Medicine, ideal digestion takes place when your stomach is no more than three-fourths full at the end of the meal. For most people, this is roughly two cupped handfuls of food. Listen to your body's signals to find out how much food you can comfortably digest, and stop eating well before you feel stuffed. When you know that you've really had enough, don't go for that second serving, no matter how tempting it is.

Don't eat before the previous meal has been digested

It takes most people about two-and-a-half hours to digest a meal. The digestive process unfolds in distinct, sequential phases. If you eat between meals, it disrupts this finely tuned process and creates ama.

Eat your main meal in the middle of the day

The digestive fire is at its peak at noontime, corresponding to the zenith of the sun. By eating your largest and heaviest meal at this time, you make sure that the digestive fire can digest it efficiently. Conversely, eat lightly at suppertime when the digestive fire is relatively low. Especially avoid cheese, meat and yogurt at night as these foods are hard to digest. Breakfast should also be a light meal. Don't skip dinner or breakfast, however, as regular meals sustain the digestive fire.

"Eat when you eat."

Eat in a settled and quiet atmosphere, with your attention on the food in front of you. Feel relaxed and happy when you eat. Enjoying light conversation with your family or friends is good for digestion. However, it's impossible to give the meal your full awareness if the television is blaring, the room is crowded and noisy, or if you're trying to read, do business, or talk on the phone. Your taste buds immediately signal the stomach to prepare proper fluids to digest the tastes you are eating. The more aware you are of your experience of eating, the better your body will be at digesting.

Always sit down to eat or drink. Use this time to really taste and appreciate the food. Standing while you eat or drink strains the digestion, which begins as soon as food enters your mouth.

Eat at a moderate pace

Eating too fast can disrupt digestion, especially if you gulp down the food without chewing it properly. Chewing your food well aids the first stage of the digestive process, in which jatharagni breaks down the food entering the stomach. Eating too slowly (meaning more than an hour-long meal) can also disrupt digestion.

Sit quietly for a few minutes after eating

If you dash out while swallowing the last bite of cake, the increased physical activity will cause blood to flow away from your stomach, interfering with your digestion. Sitting quietly for three to five minutes after a meal gives your body a chance to begin the digestive process in a normal way. It's also healthy to sit quietly for a moment before you begin your meal. This is the time when, in most cultures, people bow their heads to thank God for their food. Mind and body are intimately linked, and eating with a peaceful mind and a feeling of gratitude produces a positive influence in the whole mind-body.

Treatment of Chronic Elimination Disorders

The Ayurvedic texts explain that if digestion is normal, elimination should take place each morning on arising. Your body can then start the new day without being loaded down with yesterday's waste. Many people in our society do not know what normal elimination means, however. It's very common for people to go two or more days without having a normal bowel movement. Such chronic constipation is a sign of poor digestion, and it is implicated in many chronic diseases. Besides being a sign of a weak digestion, constipation plays a major role in disrupting digestion even further.

Constipation is related to an imbalance in Vata dosha, so if Vata predominates in your physiology, you might be more susceptible to it. Vata increases in the body after age sixty, so constipation is also more common among the elderly. Constipation is linked to an imbalance in one of the Vata subdoshas, *Apana* (discussed in Chapter 6). Apana Vata directs all downward motion in the body and governs elimination and menstrual flow. It is located in the lower pelvic area, and it influences the digestive fire and Samana Vata, a subdosha that fans the digestive fire. When

Apana Vata goes out of balance, it often causes irregularities and disorders in elimination, particularly the dryness and sluggishness of bowel functioning known as constipation.

Factors that can disrupt Apana include lack of exercise, insufficient fluid intake, and eating too much dry, rough food. Too much processed or packaged food and sticky, clogging food, such as heavy sweets and yeast breads, also aggravate Apana Vata. On the mental side, stress is a major cause of Vata disturbances in general and imbalances in Apana Vata in particular. If you suffer from constipation, a physician trained in Maharishi Vedic Medicine can help determine the specific factors that cause it and recommend ways to overcome it.

As you have seen, you can improve digestion and assimilation simply by improving your eating habits—both what you eat and how you eat it. However, poor digestion is such a critical factor in the development of chronic disease that Maharishi Vedic Medicine uses numerous other therapeutic measures to enhance digestion. In the coming chapters, you'll explore how balanced digestion can be restored through Maharishi Rejuvenation therapy, neuromuscular integration exercises, herbal supplements and a number of other natural therapies.

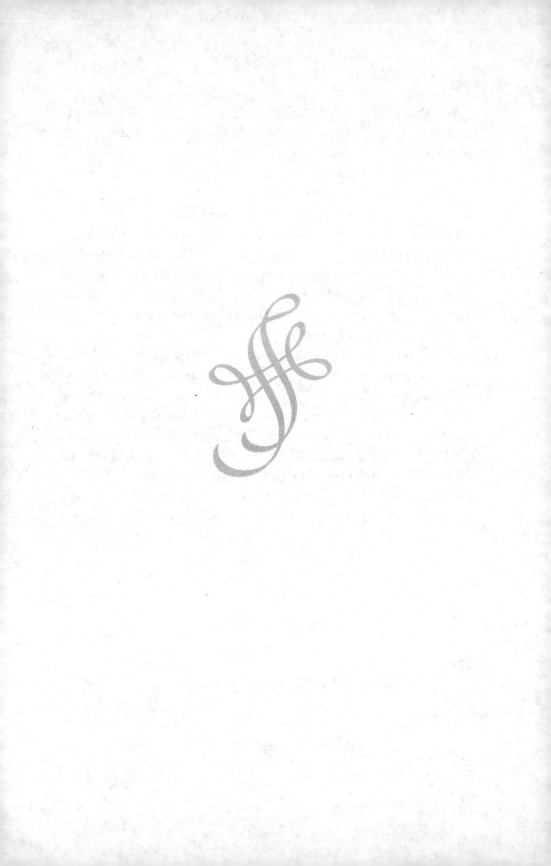

CHAPTER 16

Herbal Supplements and Rasayanas

"A person undergoing rasayana (rejuvenation) therapy attains longevity, memory, intellect, freedom from diseases, youth, excellence of luster, complexion and voice, excellent strength of the body and the sense-organs, truthful speech, respect from others, and brilliance."
—*Charaka Samhita*[42]

Harvey, a 35-year-old dentist, was suffering with his second bout of adult-onset diabetes. When he came to my office he could not keep his blood sugar level below 225 even with insulin shots. He had tried various herbal supplements and acupuncture, but his blood sugar levels stayed high.

"I knew I was in a crisis, because I felt very fragile," said Harvey. "Even eating a piece of fruit spiked my blood sugar up 100 points. I felt sluggish, weak, depressed, and at my wit's end."

I recommended a Maharishi Vedic Medicine program that included specific herbal supplements along with other treatments. Harvey found the effects of these supplements especially interesting. "Earlier tests had shown that I had insulin in my body, but I could not absorb it," he said. "The Maharishi Ayur-Veda herbs removed the toxins that were blocking the absorption of insulin." He also was also impressed with the effects of the diet I prescribed, which "seemed to enhance the healing capacity of my body."

"After about a month, maybe six weeks, I found my blood sugar was more tolerant, less out of control," Harvey said. "I felt much healthier. The treatments gave me a sense of balance and stability, and the sluggishness and depression disappeared. Now my sugar level is below ninety."

The herbal remedies have surprised me many times with their ability to awaken the body's inner healing mechanisms. For example, Monica started taking Maharishi Ayur-Veda herbal supplements along with her prescribed medication to try to balance her underactive thyroid. After about three months, she noticed that her heart was beating rapidly at night, keeping her awake. Tests showed that her thyroid had normalized. As a result, the prescribed medication was now overstimulating her system. She was eventually able to stop taking the medication altogether.

How the Herbal Compounds Are Prepared

Maharishi Ayur-Veda herbal compounds are made from a wide range of herbs prescribed in the Ayurvedic texts. They are prepared in a traditional way, according to detailed formulas and methods. These represent a sophisticated science called *dravyaguna*, literally, "qualities of matter." Anyone who studies dravyaguna must be struck by its complexity and precision. All of the Maharishi Ayur-Veda herbs are carefully formulated according to its precepts.

Although Maharishi Vedic Medicine sometimes uses single herbs, more typically it combines herbs into compounds designed to create a holistic, integrated effect. The Ayurvedic prescription for preparing both the individual herbs and the compounds emphasizes three principles:

1. **Use the whole plant, not isolated, active ingredients.** Many people, especially physicians, have become aware of the side effects of allopathic drugs. These side effects can be minimized by informed use of the whole plant. This principle contrasts directly with the modern practice of extracting the active ingredient from a plant. Western pharmacologists regularly isolate the active medicinal component in plants when they manufacture drugs,

as they believe this creates the most powerful effect. Many modern drugs are synthetic versions of the active elements in plant remedies. Aspirin, for example, was originally derived from the traditional herb known as willow bark.

A plant's active healing ingredient in its natural state actually comes wrapped in a package of other ingredients that are by no means inert. When ingested along with the active component, these seemingly incidental elements have a valuable influence. The use of a whole leaf, root, flower, or fruit, instead of a chemically extracted fragment of a plant, produces a more complete and balanced healing effect throughout the body.

2. **Employ the synergistic qualities of herbs.** Many herbal formulas prescribed by the Ayurvedic texts are based on the knowledge that certain herbs enhance each other's potency. The nutritional value of a given plant increases when incorporated with the right mixture of other herbs, because the added herbs make the nutrients and the intelligence of the plant easier for the body to assimilate. A modern term for this result is "bioavailability."

These combinations of herbs can be quite complex. One formula can involve as many as fifty herbs. The compounds usually contain a main herb, which targets the imbalance or disease. To enhance its effects, it is combined with other herbs with similar properties. Typically, at least one of these additional ingredients increases bioavailability. For example, a stimulating herb may aid absorption and assimilation of other herbs. Other herbs are generally included to help eliminate waste matter. A third type of herb may be used to balance the effects of the main herb and ensure that no imbalance is created. Finally, all the herbs together create a synergistic effect. The result is more than the sum of the parts.

The instructions for taking the herbal formula also increase its benefits. The patient is often told to take the herbal formula with a particular food or liquid, such as water, milk, ghee, or honey. These act as anupanas, or vehicles that help carry the herb to the targeted area in the cells. For example, ghee is especially useful in transporting herbal ingredients through the cell membrane, which is lipid-soluble. Anupanas can also enhance the effects of herbs or mitigate their side effects. For example, milk taken with spicy herbal formulas can help prevent those formulas from vitiating Pitta. Sometimes the anupana is contained within the herbal formula itself.

3. **Use precisely prescribed preparation methods to preserve the herb's potency and ensure that it is not damaged.** Since wild herbs are more potent than cultivated ones, many of the herbs used in Maharishi Ayur-Veda formulas are hand-gathered at their peak potency. After being collected at the correct stage of growth, the herbs are sorted to make sure that only healthy, vital herbs are used. Then the process of mixing the herbs begins.

   The science of dravyaguna gives directions for making herbal compounds in a variety of forms, each of which is most compatible with the nature and purpose of the herbal mixture. These include pastes, extracts, syrups, fresh juices, decoctions, hot infusions, cold infusions, tablets, and powders. The material for powders and tablets is first dried and crushed. Herbs for jellies and pastes must be cooked slowly for several days. Other formulas are steeped or cooked into liquids or decoctions. It can take days, sometimes even months, to process these herbs correctly.

The Balancing Effect of Herbs

In my experience with Maharishi Ayur-Veda herbal remedies, I have been particularly impressed by the fact that they create overall physiological balance at the same time that they focus on specific diseases. Each herbal formula removes impurities, balances related subdoshas, nourishes the involved dhatus, restores ojas, and awakens the body's healing intelligence.

Removes impurities

Herbs reach the cells through the minute srotas, or circulatory channels of the body. These srotas must first be purified or cleansed of obstructions. Many herbs help remove ama from the srotas. In addition, the physician often prescribes other therapies, such as an ama-reducing diet or rejuvenation treatments, to improve the body's ability to make maximum use of the herbs.

Herbs are classified according to the body's sixteen systems of srotas. Each herbal compound helps to remove impurities from one of those systems: respiratory, digestive, lymphatic, circulatory, muscular, adipose (fat), skeletal, nervous, reproductive, excretory, urinary, and sebaceous (sweat).

Balances the doshas

The three doshas operate throughout Nature, which means that they are also at work in the world of plants. For example, some plants are dry and bony and have the qualities of Vata. Others are succulent, large, and strong, and display Kapha characteristics. Pitta-dominant plants may have a reddish color and medium size and strength.

The plants also have different tastes. Some balance Vata, as they are mainly sour, sweet, or salty. Pitta-pacifying plants have astringent, bitter, or sweet properties; Kapha-pacifying herbs are bitter, astringent, or pungent. Prescribing the correct herbal mixture for the particular subdoshas that are out of balance can bring the doshas back into equilibrium and contribute significantly to the cure of disease.

Nourishes the dhatus

Herbs are also classified according to the dhatu (body tissue) that they help restore. Certain herbs help purify and build blood tissue, others bring balance to muscle tissue, while others produce strong bones or repair them. It is this specificity that allows the herbs to rejuvenate certain body tissues.

Restores ojas

Many herbal formulas help improve digestion, so that the body can eliminate ama and produce ojas, the refined by-product of healthy digestion. They strengthen agni, the digestive fire, which results in increased ojas, immunity, and overall physiological strength. Agni is also present in plants in the form of photosynthesis. Agni in plants transforms sunlight into life.

Restores wholeness

When you take herbs, you ingest the intelligence of Nature. When you take an herbal formula, you are not taking it merely for its material elements or nutritional value. You absorb the herb's intelligence, which triggers the intelligence of the body in a specific area. Ayurvedic pharmacology matches an herb's quality of intelligence or healing with the part of the mind-body that needs repair.

Rasayanas

Rasayanas, an especially valuable type of herbal compound, are designed to promote bala (strength and immunity) and ojas. The Ayurvedic texts describe two types of rasayanas: preventive and curative. The preventive rasayanas promote longevity, memory and intelligence. The curative rasayanas treat diseases.

Rasayanas also produce immunity, youthfulness, radiant skin, fertility, a clear voice and effective speech, physical strength, strong sensory perception and increased sattva (purity).

As the list suggests, rasayanas rejuvenate the mind as well as the body. "Rasayana has for its object the prolongation of human life, and the refreshment and invigoration of the memory and the vital organs of man. It deals with formulas which enable a man to retain his manhood or youthful vigor up to a good old age, and which generally serve to make the human system invulnerable to disease and decay."[43]

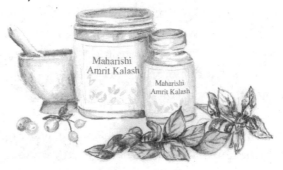

Maharishi Amrit Kalash

In Maharishi Vedic Medicine there is one rasayana that is particularly helpful in preventing and treating chronic disease called Maharishi Amrit Kalash. It is considered the king of the rasayanas because of the great range and power of its results. Modern researchers have found that this ancient elixir is extremely effective in combating a wide spectrum of diseases, including arteriosclerosis and cancer. Reports from people taking Maharishi Amrit Kalash indicate that it also reduces fatigue, combats stress, creates balance, elevates energy levels, restores inner calm, provides a sense of well-being, improves creativity and sharpens mental focus and alertness.

Combating Free Radicals

Dr. Hari Sharma, professor of pathology and director of cancer prevention and natural products research at The Ohio State University College of Medicine, conducted a series of research studies on Maharishi Amrit Kalash. He postulated that the herbal formula had so many beneficial applications—including treatment of many chronic diseases—because it was remarkably effective in eliminating free radicals.

Increasing numbers of scientists now see free radicals—which the body generates as a result of its own waste production or from toxic substances it is exposed to—as major contributors to disease and cell destruction. They are known to be neutralized by antioxidants such as vitamins A, C, and E and other nutrients. However, the antioxidant vitamins available today don't actually penetrate cell membranes—and therefore have limited ability to neutralize or "scavenge" the dangerous free radicals.

Dr. Sharma found that Maharishi Amrit Kalash is a thousand times more effective than vitamins C or E in scavenging free radicals, in part because it neutralizes a broad range of free radicals. Isolated ingredients, such as vitamin A or C, usually can only scavenge one type of free radical (see box at end of chapter).

Prescribing Herbs

Dravyaguna has many aspects besides herb preparation. How an herb is prescribed involves many considerations, including dosage, time of day and season, diagnosis of the disease or imbalance, and personal constitution. To quote the Ayurvedic texts: "Therapeutical propriety depends upon the dose of the therapy and time of administration. Success of treatment depends upon the observance of this propriety. A physician proficient in the principles of propriety is always superior to those who are acquainted with the drugs only."[46]

Prescription is a precise process, quite different from just going to a health food store and picking a few herbs off the shelf. It is essential for a person with chronic disease to seek the advice of a physician. Only a specially trained physician can accurately diagnose the specific imbalances and prescribe the correct herbal formulas to help unwind the knot of chronic disease.

Five Principles of Herbs

When preparing and prescribing herbs, the plant's taste (*rasa*), quality (*guna*), potency (*virya*), aftertaste (*vipaka*), and particular effect (*prabhava*) must all be taken into account. These five functional principles are also found in food, and are considered in determining diet.

Rasa

Rasa means essence or taste. Herbs, like food, contain the six tastes—sweet, sour, salty, pungent, bitter, astringent—in different proportions. Each taste influences the doshas, either increasing or decreasing them. Bitter, astringent and pungent herbs increase Vata. Sour, salty and pungent herbs increase Pitta. Sweet, sour and salty herbs increase Kapha.

Guna

Guna means quality. The Ayurvedic texts describe twenty qualities—heavy, cold, oily, slow, stable, soft, clear, rough, gross, semi-solid, light, hot, dry, rapid and acute, mobile, hard, viscous, smooth, subtle, and liquid. These qualities also influence the doshas. Herbs with hot, liquid, acute qualities increase Pitta; herbs with cold, oily, slow, stable, soft qualities increase Kapha; and herbs with dry, rough, hard qualities increase Vata.

Virya

The virya, or potency, of the herb is categorized as hot, cold, light, heavy, unctuous, non-unctuous, dull or sharp. The virya affects the doshas in a number of ways as it either energizes (heats) or calms (cools) the body.

Vipaka

Vipaka is the post-digestive effect, or aftertaste, of the herb.

Sometimes an herb will have a salty taste but a sweet aftertaste. Other times the taste and the aftertaste will match. Vipaka includes only three tastes, sweet, sour, or pungent.

Prabhava

Prabhava is the characteristic of an herb that makes it unique. For example, some herbs purge the body of toxins, while others nourish and build specific dhatus. Some cleanse the liver. Others strengthen the heart. This distinguishing action of an herb makes it useful in targeting specific diseases. Herbs affect the mind as well as the body. Some herbs strengthen intellect, increase mental sattva (purity), or calm the mind.

You now have a sense of both the specificity and comprehensiveness of Maharishi Ayur-Veda's knowledge of the gifts of the plant kingdom. Through the quality of their consciousness, the ancient authors of Ayurvedic texts were able to identify these healing plants and herbs and use them to reenliven the natural intelligence in cells, tissues, and organs to prevent disease and reestablish health.

Ayurveda tells us that wherever a disease exists, its cure will be found growing nearby, a principle practiced and understood by many indigenous peoples, including Native Americans. Therefore medicinal plants will vary from region to region around the globe, but the Ayurvedic principles that explain how they help us and the importance of proper preparation are universally applicable. Maharishi has placed a great emphasis on preserving regional biodiversity and indigenous knowledge because they contain a great deal of what we need to treat many of the conditions currently plaguing us. When a region's ecosystem is destroyed, many things are lost, including its vast natural pharmacy. Maharishi's revival of Ayurveda includes a concerted effort to preserve both the existence and the ancient knowledge of healing herbs and plants in every part of the world.

This chapter explained that certain herbs act best in combination with other herbs or facilitating substances. In the next chapter, you'll learn about one such application of herbs in the form of a highly beneficial oil massage, which you can easily learn to give yourself.

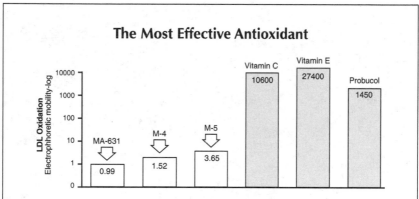

The Most Effective Antioxidant

Comparison of Different Anti-Oxidants

MA-631, M-4, M-5 vs. vitamins C, E, and probucol, p< .0001

Research shows that Maharishi Amrit Kalash is 1000 times more effective than Vitamin C in scavenging free radicals.

Reference: H.M. Sharma et al., "Inhibition of Human Low-Density Lipoprotein Oxidation in Vitro by Maharishi Amrit Kalash and Maharishi Coffee Substitute" *Pharmacology, Biochemistry and Behavior*, vol. 43 (1992), pp. 1175–1182.

Increased Resistence to Disease

Research shows that Maharishi Amrit Kalash:

- increases immunity
- prevents atherosclerosis by reducing human platelet aggregation
- reduces LDL (bad) cholesterol
- reduces chemical toxicity

References: 1. "Enhanced Lymphoproliferative Response, Macrophage-Mediated Tumor Cell Killing and Nitric Oxide Production after Ingestion of an Ayurvedic Drug (Maharishi Amrit Kalash)," *Biochemical Archives*, vol. 9 (1993), pp. 365–374.
2. H.M. Sharma et al., "Maharishi Amrit Kalash Prevents Human Platelet Aggregation," *Clinica and Terapia Cardiovascolare*, vol. 8, no. 3 (1989), pp. 227–230.
3. A.N. Hanna et al., "Effect of Herbal Mixtures MAK-4 and MAK-5 on Susceptibility of Human LDL to Oxidation, *Complementary Medicine International*, vol. 3, no. 3 (May/June 1996), pp. 28-36.
4. S.C. Bondy, et al., "Antioxidant Properties of Two Ayurvedic Herbal Preparations (MAK-4 and MAK-5)," *Biochemical Archives*, vol. 10 (1994), pp. 25-31.

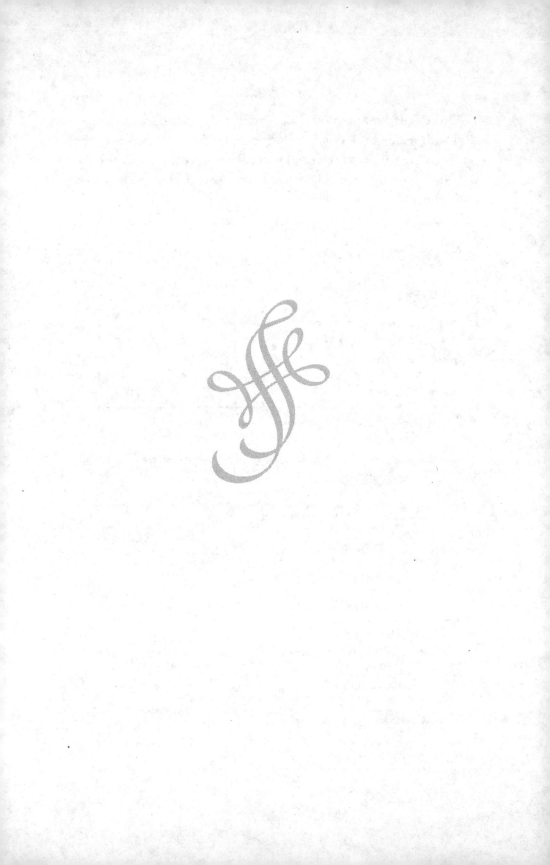

CHAPTER 17

Ayurvedic Oil Massage

"As a pitcher, a dry skin, and an axle of a cart become strong and resistant by the application of oil, so by the massage of oil the human body becomes strong and smooth-skinned; it is not susceptible to the diseases due to Vata; it is resistant to exhaustions and exertions. Vata dominates in the tactile sensory organ, and this organ is lodged in the skin. The daily oil massage is exceedingly beneficial to the skin; so one should practice it regularly. Of the one who practices oil massage regularly, the body, even if subjected to injuries or strenuous work, is not much injured; his physique is smooth, toned, strong and charming. By applying the oil massage regularly the onslaught of aging is slackened."

—*Charaka Samhita*[47]

A simple way to prevent and treat chronic disease is to start each day with an Ayurvedic oil massage, or *abhyanga*. It is usually done with warm sesame oil, which balances all three doshas. Herbs can be added to enhance the balancing effects and treat specific diseases. The warm oil soothes and calms the whole body. Though sesame oil is recommended for most people, coconut or olive oil might be prescribed for individuals with sensitive skin, depending on the predominant dosha.

Morning is the best time for the massage, and it takes ten to fifteen minutes. Many people find that abhyangas gently get them ready for the day without having to take harmful stimulants such as coffee. Others notice that they feel more energetic and alert, ready to face the day's challenges with greater ease. It also tones and cleanses the skin, restoring its youthful and elastic qualities.

The Benefits of Ayurvedic Oil Massage

Abhyanga relieves a variety of conditions, including the following:

Joint stiffness	Poor circulation
Fatigue	Poor immunity
Dryness	Vata imbalance
Poor muscle tone	Cellulite
Physical and mental exhaustion	Sleep disorders

I have seen this simple technique dramatically improve the health of many of my patients. Dianne, a 55-year-old grandmother, was experiencing classical menopausal problems. She had hot flashes, headaches, insomnia, and a general overall feeling of discomfort.

"I was working for an HMO," she said, "but the medical doctors seemed to pooh-pooh my problems. I knew I had to do something else, because I was getting nowhere with the conventional approach."

Diane started a series of Maharishi Vedic Medicine treatments, and within three months she noticed a major shift in her symptoms.

"I feel 90 per cent better," she said. "I think all of the approaches helped—the herbal supplements, the diet, and the exercise. I do the abhyanga every day. I think it definitely stimulates the body and circulation, and creates more wakefulness in the morning. I just feel great when I do that. My day starts out very, very well. I have more energy. My emotional state is happy and calm.

"Maharishi Vedic Medicine offers some wonderful approaches that work. And your body starts functioning as it should, using its own resources. Anyone can learn how to do it. It also has the advantage of being very inexpensive, especially when you compare it to the yield in improved health and relief from many chronic ailments."

Improved Immunity and Detoxification

For the chronically ill patient, Ayurvedic oil massage is a simple but powerful way to improve bala, or immunity. The skin is the largest organ in the body, and all the body's organs have nerve endings connected to the skin. When you stimulate the skin, you are in a sense stimulating every organ in the body, helping to flush out toxins and rejuvenate all the internal organs.

Warm oil massage also increases immunity by clearing away toxins and blockages from the srotas. The toxins flow into the alimentary tract, where the body's elimination system moves them out through the urine or bowels. When the srotas are clear, more nutrition can reach each cell, and each cell can dispose of its waste products more efficiently. Ama is removed and ojas, the body's natural healing intelligence, can flow throughout the body unimpeded.

The removal of toxins even takes place in the cell membranes, which are composed of lipids, or fatty molecules. The fresh massage oil penetrates the skin's layers and replaces the old, toxin-filled molecules in the cell membranes. It flushes out the cell walls by replacing the old fatty molecules with new, fresh, fatty molecules.

Balanced Doshas

Touch is associated with Vata, which is dry and cool, so the warm oil counteracts any imbalance in Vata. The massage strokes also help calm Vata by soothing the skin. Vata leads the other doshas. When Vata is balanced, it helps keep all the doshas balanced, which in turn supports prevention. For someone who is sick, abhyanga's powerful balancing effect assists healing.

Gentle touch with the intention of healing brings harmony to your entire body and enlivens its inner healing intelligence. When you focus your consciousness on your body through touch, you help maintain (or reestablish) the vital mind-body connection.

How to Do an Ayurvedic Oil Massage

The ideal time for an abhyanga is just before you bathe or shower in the morning. Most people should use cold-pressed sesame oil, preferably organic. Cold-pressed sesame oil is available at health food stores. (To order organic sesame oil, or dosha-specific herbalized oils, see the information in the Appendix.) Create an application system that will put the oil on you, not your floor or furniture. Some people perform the massage in an empty bathtub. Others cut a plastic garbage bag, spread it on the floor, and cover it with a sheet, which they can launder regularly.

Prepare the oil by curing it before you use it. (Instructions for curing are given below.) Heat the oil to a comfortable temperature. It should warm, not burn. Many people put the cured oil in a small, flip-top plastic bottle and immerse it in warm water.

Use the open part of your hand, rather than your finger tips, to massage your entire body. In general, use circular motions over rounded areas (joints, face) and straight strokes over straight areas (neck, arms, legs and back). Apply moderate pressure over most of your body and light pressure over your abdomen and heart. Vata and Pitta-dominant people should stroke toward the heart, while Kaphic people should stroke away from it.

1. Start with your head. Pour a small amount of warm oil on your hands and vigorously massage it into your scalp. Using the flat part of your hands, make circular strokes to cover your whole head. Spend more time massaging your head than other parts of your body.
2. Move to your face and outer ears, applying a small amount of oil. Massage this area more gently.
3. Massage the front and back of your neck, and the upper part

of your spine. At this point, cover the rest of your body with a small layer of oil to give it maximum time to soak in.

4. Vigorously massage your arms, using a circular motion on your shoulders and elbows (front and back) and long, back-and-forth strokes on your upper arms and forearms.

5. Massage your chest and stomach area, using a light, circular motion over your heart and abdomen. You can start in the lower right part of your abdomen and move clockwise toward the left lower part, to gently massage your intestines.

6. Massage your back and spine as far as you can comfortably reach.

7. Massage your legs vigorously, using circular motions over your hips, knees and ankles. Use long, straight strokes over your thighs and calves.

8. Finally, massage the bottoms of your feet. As with your head, you can spend more time on this important area. Use the palm of your hand to massage the soles vigorously, and cover every area.

9. Follow your oil massage with a warm bath or shower.

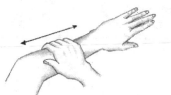

This massage is not only healthy but also luxurious and relaxing. It energizes and stimulates every organ and simultaneously tones and revitalizes your skin. It increases strength and immunity, detoxifies, and gently dissolves the lethargy of sleep. What a perfect way to start the day.

Curing Sesame Oil

Maharishi Vedic Medicine recommends "cured," unprocessed, cold-pressed sesame oil. To cure the oil, place up to one quart in a saucepan and heat it to the boiling temperature of water. (You don't need to boil the oil, as that could be dangerous.) Use a candy thermometer to monitor the heat constantly. *As the oil begins to heat, the temperature will begin to rise more quickly, so watch it very carefully.* Once the temperature reaches 212 degrees Fahrenheit, the oil is cured and you should immediately remove it from the heat and place it on a cool surface, such as in your sink or on a hot pad on your countertop, out of the reach of children. The whole curing process takes only about five minutes.

You can cure up to one quart of oil at a time. This should be enough for at least two weeks.

Because all oils are flammable, be sure to observe proper safety precautions. (Your kitchen should naturally be equipped with a chemical fire extinguisher; also, a tight-fitting lid can help smother a small oil fire.) Use low rather than high heat and never leave the room while the oil is heating. Be sure to keep it out of the reach of children while it cools off.

CHAPTER 18

Daily Routine: Synchronizing Physiological Rhythms with the Rhythms of Nature

"As life is a continuum of smaller and bigger cycles, it is necessary to consider health not only in terms of isolated, specific points, but also in terms of cycles. It is the cycles that constitute the breath of life, which is always moving in an evolutionary direction."

—*Maharishi Mahesh Yogi*[48]

By the time Susan came to me, she was desperate. A 41-year-old hairstylist, she suffered from severe digestive problems which created painful gas, bloating, and severe constipation. This was accompanied by continuous hot flashes and night sweats, which had left her sleepless for months at a time. Fatigue, mental stress, and mood swings added to her discomfort. Medications for her digestive problems and for depression brought little relief. She complained of a rapid heartbeat, which she identified as a side effect of the medication.

In less than one month of treatment, which included changes in her daily routine, Susan's hot flashes disappeared completely. Her headache, insomnia, digestive disorders, and constipation also improved. As a result, her depression and mood swings abated and she was able to stop taking the antidepressant and digestive medications. Her heartbeat is now normal and she has energy for the first time in years.

She wrote, "I can't believe that something could work as rapidly as Maharishi Vedic Medicine. I also liked being given lifestyle changes, rather than being told, 'take the medicine and go eat and do whatever you want.' I like it that Maharishi Vedic Medicine offers a whole way of living that's healthy."

The relationship between behavior and health is now well-established. Everyone knows that high-risk behaviors such as smoking can destroy health over time.

Ayurvedic texts have emphasized for centuries that lifestyle is among the most important determinants of health or disease. Based on millennia of experience, Maharishi Vedic Medicine gives detailed advice on important aspects of routine and lifestyle that are, at best, just beginning to gain attention in Western medicine.

Biorhythms are one such aspect. Medical research has begun to look at the body's daily, monthly, and annual biological cycles to learn how they affect health. Scientists have discovered that the dosages of certain medications must be adjusted according to the time of day they are administered. However, Maharishi Vedic Medicine goes much further. It has long recognized the crucial role of biorhythms in maintaining strong immunity and vibrant health overall. Daily routine—when you wake up, sleep, eat, and so forth—actually makes an enormous difference both in the short and long term.

Physiological cycles are attuned to the natural patterns of the planet on which we live. For thousands of years, your ancestors rose and retired with the sun. Only in the last century or so, with the advent of electric lighting, have people been able to choose when to wake up or go to sleep and to separate themselves from the natural rhythms of night and day. As wonderful as that freedom may seem, its abuse has taken its toll on health. Your body simply was not designed to run continuously on late nights and too little sleep. It was designed to rise and retire with the sun.

Putting Health in Your Schedule

Following an optimal daily routine produces definite rewards. When you align your biorhythms with the rhythms of Nature, you tap into Nature's infinite energy and orderliness. Rather than fighting against your body and its innate cycles, you start using them to create health and energy. Many of my patients significantly improved their health just by changing some habits. A few adjustments can make a big difference. Attune your waking and sleeping cycle to Nature to help correct imbalances and heal sleep disorders. Eat your main meal at noon when agni is at its peak, and your digestive strength will increase. Other benefits include increased energy, less fatigue and lethargy, balanced doshas, stronger agni, reduced ama and toxins, and reduced stress.

When to wake up, when to sleep, when to eat. There is a natural time of day for every important function. Just as it's easier to flow with the current of a river than to paddle against it, following a life-supporting daily routine is quite easy, because your body wants to follow its natural rhythms.

The Three Basic Rhythms of Vata, Pitta, and Kapha

The doshas provide a useful window on natural cycles. As explained in Chapter 5, each dosha governs different hours in the day. In the early evening, as darkness falls, everything seems to slow down and feel heavier, quieter. This corresponds to Kapha dosha, which is heavy and slow. Contrast this with sunrise, when the birds burst into song, embodying the active, vital feeling of the new day. This time of day reflects the qualities of Vata—active, moving, full of energy. When the sun rises high in the sky at noon, hot Pitta dosha dominates.

As you become more aware of the daily cycles of Vata, Pitta, and Kapha, you will find yourself automatically doing the things that bring balance to your mind and body. To foster that awareness,

Maharishi Vedic Medicine offers many specific guidelines for alining with Nature's cycles and creating optimal health.

The daily routine is divided into three sections: morning, midday, and evening. Let's look at the details of each.

Wake Up with Alertness: The Morning Routine

Some people feel groggy in the morning and continue to feel groggy all day. Some people think it's normal to wake up feeling tired. In many cases, this is due to unnatural sleep habits. As you start to follow the Ayurvedic routine of early to bed and early to rise and begin to experience more balance in your mind and body, you'll find yourself waking up feeling increasingly light and buoyant.

The morning routine has its real foundation in the preceding evening. Retire before 10 p.m. if possible. After going to bed early and getting enough sleep, it is easier to fulfill the first morning recommendation of Maharishi Vedic Medicine. Get up before 6 a.m., which is when the morning Kapha cycle starts. The evening Kapha cycle (6–10 p.m.) is optimum for falling asleep. The morning Kapha cycle (6–10 a.m.), on the other hand, is not a good time for waking up. If you rise during the morning Kapha period, your mind-body gets suffused with the dull, slow, heavy qualities of Kapha, and you may feel these influences throughout the day. Maharishi Vedic Medicine recommends that you wake up with the birds, while Vata dominates, to benefit from its light, energizing qualities.

Getting up early and at the same time every day, regardless of what time you went to bed, is one of the most important steps to getting in tune with Nature's rhythms. The logic for this is simple: If you get up consistently early over a few days or weeks, you will start to feel sleepy earlier in the evening, and you will soon be falling asleep at a healthy hour.

The Ayurvedic Oil Massage (Abhyanga)

This special, full-body massage with warm sesame oil is a key element of the Ayurvedic daily routine.

Bathing

After your abhyanga, wash off the sesame oil in a warm bath or shower. Warm water helps open the srotas so that impurities loosened through massage can flow into the elimination system.

Cleaning the Mouth

You probably are already accustomed to cleaning your teeth first thing in the morning. The Ayurvedic texts mention using special twigs to clean teeth. The toothbrush and dental floss are modern equivalents. It's also important to clean your tongue in the morning by scraping it with a special tongue scraper made of silver or other metals. Ama collects on the surface of the tongue. You may have noticed it as a whitish coating. When you gently remove this film of impurities from your tongue each morning, you help to purify your colon and improve digestion.

Another important part of the Ayurvedic wake-up routine is gargling with warm sesame oil. Sesame oil gargle (*gandusha*) and sesame oil gum massage can help protect your mouth from harmful bacteria and gum deterioration. Edwards Smith, M.D., and scientists at The Wichita State University's College of Health Professionals found that swishing oil in the mouth and then gargling with sesame oil significantly reduced the number of species of bacteria in the space between teeth and gums.[49] Researchers consider bacteria in this area to be the major cause of gum disease. In addition, since gandusha strengthens and purifies the entryway for food—the mouth, where the initial steps of digestion take place—it also improves digestion.

"Gargling is beneficial for the strength of jaws, depth of voice, facial skin tone, excellent gustatory sensation, and good taste for food. One who is used to such gargles never gets dryness of throat, nor do his lips ever get cracked; his teeth will never have cavities and will be deep-rooted; he will not have any toothache nor will his teeth be set on edge by sour intake; his teeth can chew even the hardest eatables."[50]

Instructions for Gandusha

Gandusha is traditionally done in the morning after the abhyanga. Use fresh, warm sesame oil that has been cured. (See Chapter 17 for curing instructions.)

1. Fill your mouth as fully as comfort allows with warm sesame oil. Hold the oil in your mouth for thirty to sixty seconds, then let it out.

2. Repeat Step 1.

3. Take a little warm oil in your mouth and gargle for thirty to sixty seconds. Let it out.

4. Massage the oil into your gums with your finger. Be gentle, but use enough pressure for the massage to be pleasantly invigorating. Take two or three minutes to do this thoroughly.

5. If you wish, you can rinse your mouth with warm water to remove any oily residue.

Maharishi Yoga Asanas

These neuromuscular integration exercises are special postures that help remove toxins and enliven vital points of the body. They also help reduce stress and fatigue and prepare your body for meditation.

Yoga means "union," and refers to the union of mind and body. The word asana means "established." In this usage, it means "established in the Self, or pure consciousness." Asanas help connect each part of the body to its source in the Self, enlivening the flow of consciousness in every cell. Asanas are useful in treating chronic disease because they create mental and physical stability, improve mind-body coordination, increase circulation, and create both flexibility and strength. Specific asanas enliven and rejuvenate different organs, glands, and physiological systems: One pose may strengthen the digestive system, while another may strengthen the lungs. Maharishi Vedic Medicine physicians may therefore prescribe specific asanas. Maharishi Vedic University also offers a sixteen-lesson course on a comprehensive set of asanas that can be done regularly.

Surya Namaskara

A special set of asanas, or neuromuscular integration exercises, the *Surya Namaskara* ("salute to the sun") is particularly helpful for digestion and elimination. It strengthens all the muscles in the body and helps create deeper integration of body and mind.

Neurorespiratory Integration Exercises (Pranayama)

These simple, rhythmic breathing exercises produce balanced, relaxed breathing and vitalizing energy throughout the mind-body. *Pranayama* purifies and refines the life breath (Prana), brings oxygen to the cells, and clears the srotas. When done before meditation, it helps calm the mind and remove surface stress. It is especially helpful for purifying and relaxing the lungs.

The Transcendental Meditation *Technique*

You have already read in Chapter 12 about this important part of the daily routine. This simple technique is the foundation for all Maharishi Vedic Medicine approaches, because it settles and expands the mind and removes stress from the body. It is the most important thing you can do to prepare for the day and align yourself with Nature.

Feel Energetic All Day: The Midday Routine

If possible, choose a profession or course of study that supports your doshic makeup. If you are predominantly Vata, for example, try to find work that makes you feel settled, rather than scattered or pressured. A job involving much travel would aggravate Vata. If you have a Kapha imbalance, on the other hand, you may need a certain amount of stimulation and excitement to counteract your tendency to feel inert or complacent. For Pitta-dominant people, too much pressure or competition on the job, as well as working in the hot sun, increase Pitta.

Eat your main meal at noon. When the sun is at its zenith, agni, the digestive fire, is also at its peak. If you eat your heaviest meal at noon, you'll process it more efficiently and find it easier to eat lightly at night. After eating, sit quietly for a few minutes and then take a brief walk to aid digestion. Following these suggestions will improve your health and help you be more alert and effective in your afternoon's activities.

Fall Asleep Easily at Night: The Evening Routine

Nearly every physician tells his or her patients, "Try to get more rest." When the body is ailing, deep rest is part of the cure. It is during sleep that the body repairs itself. If you suffer from chronic disease, you need more rest than other people.

Maharishi Vedic Medicine places great importance on sleep. It is considered one of the pillars of health in Vedic texts, on par with diet and the TM technique.[51] Unfortunately, contemporary society has a rampant problem with insomnia and interrupted sleep. In a recent survey, the great majority of those interviewed said that they did not get enough sleep at night. Insomnia, a disease characterized by the inability to sleep even when exhausted, afflicts fifty million Americans. Insomnia is also implicated in many other chronic diseases, either as a contributing factor or as a by-product.

Sleep disorders can be caused by imbalances in Pitta or Vata dosha. Vata disorders can cause difficulty in falling asleep, while

Pitta disorders can cause restless and broken sleep. Both of these imbalances can be helped by going to bed early, when Kapha dominates, which means before 10 p.m. During this period (6 to 10 p.m.), Kapha's heavy, dull, stable qualities facilitate falling asleep. When you fall asleep at this time, sleep is deeper and more restful.

If you stay awake past 10:00, when the evening Pitta cycle starts (10 p.m. to 2 a.m.), you naturally begin to feel more energetic and it is more difficult to fall asleep. Sleep takes on the focused, alert quality of Pitta dosha and is less restful than sleep that starts during the Kapha period before 10 p.m. Staying awake during Pitta time also tends to make you feel hungry, yet eating late at night is not a good idea. The digestive fire is very low at night and the body needs this time to rest and repair itself, and cleanse the srotas of ama. Eating after 10 p.m. produces digestive imbalance and therefore ama accumulation. It is especially important for someone with chronic disease to go to bed before 10, not only to get deeper sleep but also to rebalance the body.

Recommendations for the Nighttime Routine

Eat only a light meal in the evening, and eat before 8 p.m. Eating lightly at night is better for digestion and results in better sleep.

Save the evening hours for quiet, relaxing activities. Even watching TV before bed can aggravate Vata and disturb your sleep. If you do watch TV, try to turn it off before 9 p.m. Instead, listen to music, visit with friends, and spend time with your family.

Terry, a 48-year-old radiologist with Vata and Pitta imbalances, found that following the complete Ayurvedic routine helped him sleep more deeply. Previously, he went to bed late (after 11:30 p.m.) and ate at all different times of the day. He woke up for long periods in the night, tossing and turning. In the morning, he drank three cups of coffee just to wake up, and then he felt hyper all day.

After starting the Ayurvedic routine, Terry started going to bed at 10 p.m., avoided working at night, and began eating regular meals. His sleep problems cleared up. He stopped waking up in the night and slept deeply until morning. "After being on the routine for about six months, I noticed that I was no longer using an alarm clock to wake up at 5:30," he said. "Now I wake up naturally around 4:45 or 5:00. I had been wondering how I was going to fit in the whole morning routine, but I then I noticed I was sleeping less than I was originally. I also noticed that in the afternoon I still felt good, whereas before I felt tired. I was more calm at work and able to handle the emergencies and stressful times better. I felt more in charge and less at the mercy of the workload. Now I am more alert and awake, and that makes me more effective in activity.

"I no longer have any need for coffee. The daily Ayurvedic oil massage makes me feel awake, but not nervous—just the opposite feeling of coffee, which makes me feel more nervous than awake. I feel more energetic, and less worried and irritable all day."

As you can see from Terry's story, going to bed early and doing the wake-up routine produces benefits all day.

Exercise

Some people want more physical exercise than the Maharishi Yoga asanas and Surya Namaskara provide. Exercise is certainly a part of the Ayurvedic routine. The Ayurvedic texts mention that correct exercise "makes the body light and glossy, firm and compact; banishes fatigue and weariness; makes the body strong and helps the symmetrical growth of the limbs and muscles; aids in enduring variations of temperature, thirst, etc.; leads to an existence without disease; stimulates the power of digestion, alleviates the doshas, makes an aged and deformed person look young and good looking; improves complexion, and prevents laziness."[52]

Exercise is an effective way to flush toxins out of the body and infuse the cells with oxygen. It is certainly important for maintaining health. As mentioned in Chapter 5, inactivity is potentially a cause of disease.

The Ayurvedic guidelines for exercise prohibit getting fatigued or exhausted. The proper intensity, speed, and duration depends on individual capacity, imbalances, and constitutional type. For many people, especially those who have more of the active Vata dosha, asanas and Surya Namaskaras, along with half an hour of walking, is enough. For others, especially those with more of the slower, more phlegmatic Kapha dosha, vigorous exercise is needed to stay healthy. Indeed, your choice of exercise can help balance all three doshas.

Guidelines for Healthy Exercise

In some chronic diseases, such as hypertension, vigorous exercise may be dangerous. Before beginning any exercise program, consult your primary physician.

The optimum time to exercise is during the morning Kapha period. This is when the body is strongest and when exercise has the most beneficial effect, as it clears out the heaviness of the night's sleep. If you can't exercise then, the next best time is the afternoon, although not right after lunch. Never exercise on a full stomach. Exercise can interfere with digestion, so wait two hours after a meal to exercise. Before a meal, allow half an hour to recover from exercise before eating.

Exercise every day for about half an hour. The body needs to stretch and move daily as part of your regular routine.

Use only 50 per cent of your capacity when you exercise. The "no pain, no gain" philosophy has no part in Maharishi Vedic Medicine. Stop before you are tired, rather than pushing yourself to the limit. If you can walk ten miles before feeling exhausted, then stop at five. If you exercise daily and stay within your zone of ease, you will naturally increase your capability over time without any strain on the body. You should never feel tired or exhausted after exercising—only invigorated. Weariness is a sign of excessive exercise and should be avoided at all costs, especially if you are combating a disease.

Maharishi Yoga Asanas and Surya Namaskara are excellent exercises for almost everybody. This includes people of all three constitutional types and for many people with chronic disease. (Check with your physician to make sure.) Likewise, a daily walk in fresh air benefits almost everyone and has a positive effect on many diseases.

If your Maharishi Vedic Medicine physician feels that you need more physical activity than asanas and a thirty-minute daily walk provide, he or she will recommend exercise that is healthy for your body type. As explained earlier, Vata-dominant people need relatively light, easy exercise. People with more Pitta require exercise that is moderate in quantity and intensity. People with Kapha imbalances need longer and more intense periods of exercise.

Here are some specific examples of exercise that are particularly well suited for different constitutions:

Vata—walking, Yoga, light dance

Pitta—swimming, bicycling, tennis, weight lifting

Kapha—team sports, aerobics, jogging

The combined elements of the daily routine have a powerful influence on health. People who have followed this routine over a period of years report that their diet and lifestyle changes have generated not only freedom from disease but also continuous expansion of energy, vitality, and well-being.

Dinacharya
The Ayurvedic Daily Routine

Morning

Wake up early, before 6:00 a.m.

Evacuate your bowels and bladder.

Brush your teeth and scrape your tongue.

Gargle with sesame oil.

Give yourself an Ayurvedic oil massage.

Bathe or shower.

Do Maharishi Yoga Asanas, Surya Namaskara, and breathing techniques.

Practice the Transcendental Meditation technique.

Exercise.

Eat a light breakfast.

Midday

Work or study.

Eat your largest meal of the day between 12:00 and 1:00 p.m.

Sit quietly for a few minutes after eating.

Take a brief walk to aid digestion. Those with severely limited capacity shouldn't strain, but even 50–100 steps will be helpful.

Exercise. (Wait at least two hours after meals for strenuous exercise.)

Evening

Do Maharishi Yoga Asanas, Surya Namaskara, and breathing techniques in the late afternoon or early evening.

Practice the Transcendental Meditation technique.

Eat an early, light supper.

Sit quietly for a few minutes after eating.

Take a brief walk to aid digestion.

Enjoy light, relaxing activities.

Go to sleep before 10:00 p.m.

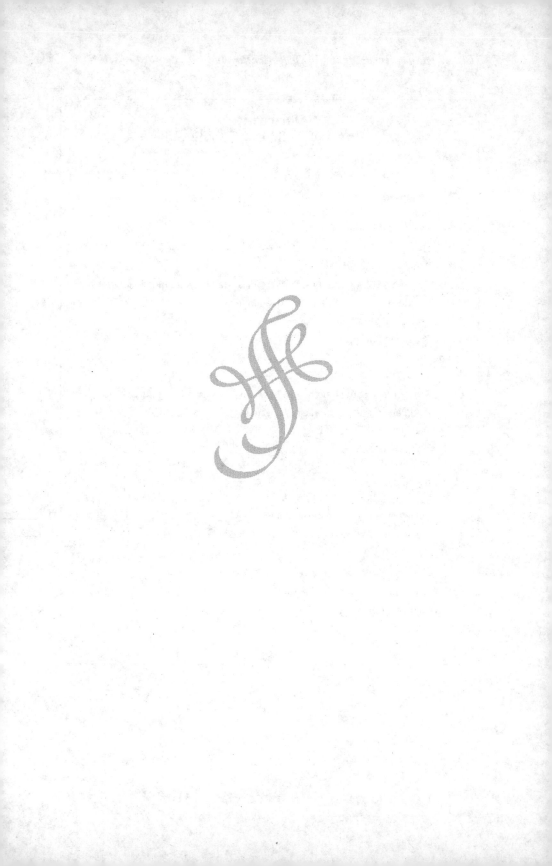

CHAPTER 19

Living in Harmony with the Seasons

"The strength and luster of one who knows the suitable diet and regimen for every season and practices accordingly are enhanced."   —*Charaka Samhita*[53]

Maharishi Vedic Medicine considers the environment to be a major factor in health care. The subtle effects of climatic conditions and even the geography of the land are considered in the diagnosis and treatment of disease.

The cycle of the seasons is a major player in your health. Vata, for example, dominates late fall and winter, which is called Vata season. It is cold, dry, and windy. In summer, or Pitta season, the sun is visible for long hours each day and its more direct rays create more heat. The rainy, cool weather in spring makes it Kapha season.

The seasons described here are common for much of North America but vary in other locations. India, for example, has six distinct seasons, but the overall rhythm of the doshas remains constant.

How the Seasons Affect Your Health

In many parts of North America and Europe, people experience extreme shifts in weather conditions as the seasons change. Even in the more temperate zones, intense summer heat can cause its own kinds of imbalances. It's important to understand that when a dosha is predominant during a particular season, the same dosha stirs inside you. You are so intimately connected with Nature that your body will mirror the changes in the weather. In the cold, dry Vata season, for example, you may find that you're too restless to fall asleep at night. Your skin and hair may become dry and itchy, or you may get constipated due to internal dryness. Many people also feel more anxious and worried in winter due to the strength of Vata dosha. In the cool, wet Kapha season, you might feel lethargic or heavy. Your digestion may be slow, and you might gain a few extra pounds. Bronchial asthma, flu, sinus congestion, and allergies flare up in the spring. Summer brings a set of potential Pitta-related problems such as hyperacidity, skin rashes, acne, hypertension, excessive thirst, hay fever, headaches, and irritability.

Seasonal Rhythms of Vata, Pitta, and Kapha (for North America)

Dosha	Doshic Quality	Corresponding Season
Kapha	cool, moist	Spring (March–June)
Pitta	hot, humid	Summer (July–October)
Vata	cold, dry, windy	Winter (November–February)

Health Routines for the Three Ayurvedic Seasons

To counteract the effects of the doshas accumulating in each season, Maharishi Vedic Medicine gives specific guidelines called *ritucharya*, or the seasonal routine. Ritucharya is based on the idea that adjustments to diet and lifestyle can reduce the physiological effects of a season's dominant dosha. During Pitta season, for example, consuming cool food and liquids will diminish Pitta in your body. In Kapha season, if you exercise more, avoid daytime naps, and eat warm, light, dry food—this will balance heavy, cold Kapha dosha. During the winter, you can balance Vata by keeping a regular routine and eating oily, heavy, warm foods which counteract light, changeable, cold Vata dosha.

The *Charaka Samhita* explains, "The experts in the subject advise habitual use of such diets [including herbal supplements] and regimen having opposite qualities of the habitat of the individuals [seasons] and the diseases they are suffering from."[54] You may already do this naturally. Here are some more examples of things you can do to decrease the accumulation of the doshas in different seasons.

Vata Season (Winter): November to February

These suggestions will balance the qualities of Vata (quick, cold, rough dry, restless, anxious), which increases in strength in winter.

Diet

- Emphasize warm foods and liquids and sweet foods such as milk, cream, wheat products, rice, sweet and ripe fruits. Favor raw sugar (in moderation) as your sweetener.
- Favor sour foods (e.g., lemons), salty foods, and heavy, oilier foods.
- Eat less of the following: astringent or dry foods (beans, broccoli, cauliflower, apples and pears); bitter foods (romaine lettuce, endive, spinach, and other leafy greens); pungent foods (chili peppers or cayenne); cold food and drinks; any food with light, dry, rough qualities. Cooking the dry vegetables such as broccoli in ghee, or mixing them with foods of a sweeter or more unctuous nature, allows you to eat them in moderate quantities.
- Emphasize these spices: cardamom, cumin, ginger, cinnamon, salt, cloves, saffron, and small quantities of black pepper.
- Milk is ideal for balancing Vata, especially when it is warm. To make milk easier to digest, avoid drinking it with a full meal. Milk is also more digestible if you add a slice of ginger and bring it to a boil before drinking it.

Daily Routine

- Start your day with a warm, luxurious Ayurvedic oil massage.
- Get lots of rest, and go to bed extra early.
- Keep warm and avoid drafts.
- Maintain a regular schedule.
- Use a humidifier to avoid winter dryness.
- Exercise moderately. Use indoor equipment if it's too cold outside.
- Drink plenty of warm liquids, such as Vata® tea, throughout the day. [See Appendix for ordering seasonal teas]

Kapha Season (Spring): March to June

More exercise and a light diet will counterbalance the heavy, cool, moist qualities of Kapha, which increases in the spring. Kapha accumulation can produce lethargy, or even a little depression, as well as hay fever, coughs, and sinus headaches.

Diet

- Emphasize warm soups, cooked foods, and spices; light, fresh foods (salads and cooked vegetables); dry foods (dahl, beans, barley, crackers); hot liquids such as Kapha® tea or ginger tea; bitter, astringent, and pungent foods.
- Cut back on oily, deep-fried food; heavy food (cheese, yogurt, ice cream); cold food and drinks; sweet, sour, and salty food.
- Avoid sugar, but uncooked honey, which is slightly astringent actually reduces Kapha. Be careful not to cook honey, as this makes it toxic.

Daily Routine

- Exercise every day. This will increase circulation, counteract Kapha's heaviness, and eliminate impurities.
- Spend some time in the morning sun when the sun is not as

harsh. Don't overdo it, though, and be sure to protect your skin.

- Cover your head and throat when it's windy.
- Avoid sleeping late or taking a nap during the day.

Pitta Season (Summer): June to October

Prevent problems associated with Pitta accumulation in the summer—heat rashes, ulcers, irritability—by following these guidelines.

Diet

- Eat less. Digestion naturally slows down in warm weather, so you'll feel healthier if you eat more lightly.
- Emphasize cool food and drinks. However, avoid ice-cold or carbonated drinks, as these inhibit digestion.
- Emphasize fresh, organic food and pure water; sweet food (milk, cream, wheat products, rice, sweet and ripe fruits); sweeteners such as raw sugar (in moderation); astringent or dry foods (beans, split-mung dahl, broccoli, cauliflower, apples, pears, pomegranates); bitter foods (romaine lettuce, endive, spinach, leafy greens).
- Reduce oily, heavy food; sour food (yogurt, sour cream, cheese, tomatoes, vinegar, sour grapes); pungent or hot food (chili pepper, salsa, cayenne, ginger, onions and garlic); salty food.
- Add cooling spices and herbs to your food and drinks such as anise, cardamom, cinnamon, coriander, cilantro, fennel, fenugreek, licorice, mint and turmeric. Drink Pitta® tea.

Daily Routine

- Exercise less and choose milder exercise to avoid getting overheated. Favor the early morning for exercising, or enjoying an evening walk in the cool moonlight. Cooling sports such as swimming are ideal.

- Protect yourself from the sun. Wear a hat and sunglasses and use sunscreen. Avoid sunbathing for long periods and avoid the noonday sun altogether.
- Keep the temperature cool when you're indoors.
- Take it easy in summer. It's the season to relax and enjoy Nature's beauty.

Lassi and Ghee

Although most oils increase Pitta, ghee (clarified butter) has a unique ability to stimulate digestion and cool Pitta at the same time. Ghee is cherished in Maharishi Vedic Medicine as a nutritional food for all body types. It doesn't burn at high temperatures, so it makes a great cooking oil. It also makes an excellent butter substitute for sandwiches or toast.

Yogurt is a sour food you generally want to avoid in summer. However, when blended with water and a sweetener, it becomes a healthy, cooling drink called lassi. Always use freshly made yogurt to prepare lassi.

Seasonal Checkups

Because the doshas are constantly fluctuating with the seasons, seasonal checkups are recommended to prevent impurities from building up. That way diet, daily routine, and your home health care program can constantly be adjusted to eliminate imbalances that have built up from the previous season, and to address your own unique constitution and circumstances. You can also receive an extensive program of purification treatments to cleanse the entire body of toxins at the end of each season.

These purification therapies, together called Maharishi Rejuvenation therapy, are the subject of the next chapter. Taking these treatments during the change of seasons is an excellent way to prevent imbalances. Maharishi Rejuvenation therapy balances doshas that have become aggravated in the previous season. It also clears the srotas of ama and allows herbal compounds and rasayanas to work more effectively in nourishing, strengthening, and revitalizing the dhatus. By following a seasonal diet and routine, and by taking Maharishi Rejuvenation therapy on a seasonal basis throughout life, you can delay the aging process, promote longevity and youthfulness, and ensure the optimum use of the senses.

CHAPTER 20

Rejuvenation Therapy

"Considering health, people generally are not aware that the physiology accumulates different kinds of toxins in the different seasons. Before a season ends, such as summer or winter, the toxins accumulated during that season must be eliminated so the body does not continue with the toxins of the previous seasons into the next season.

"There are many other things to do for good health—daily routine, proper diet, exercise—but this seasonal purification is the key to eliminate the basis of disease. If the accumulated toxins are released during each season, more than 70 per cent of the diseases will disappear on earth."   —*Maharishi Mahesh Yogi*[55]

At 45, Donna had the energy to run two businesses, handle the family finances, cook and do the housework, enjoy her grandchildren, and take care of her aging parents—all at the same time. "I was an eager beaver, a hard worker, and I enjoyed my work," said Donna. "And I thought nothing of working seventy hours a week in addition to my responsibilities at home."

When Donna started to feel fatigue and depression, she knew something was terribly wrong. The day came when she didn't even have the energy to get dressed after her shower. "I had to sit down for an hour or two to rest. I just felt lousy." Her doctor could find nothing wrong, and prescribed an antidepressant, which she didn't take.

She started to cough incessantly. Four rounds of antibiotics didn't seem to help. She also suffered from severe heartburn, constipation, and pain throughout her body. Her left leg and arm felt numb. "I'd plant a few tulips and feel like I just ran a marathon," she said. "I'd sweat, get red in the face, and feel completely out of breath."

Finally, after a year and a half of visiting doctors, a pulmonary specialist recommended a CAT scan of her lungs. A surgeon gave her the diagnosis of idiopathic pulmonary fibrosis—scarring of the lungs. He said it was idiopathic, meaning the cause was unknown. The scarring could be caused by stomach acids associated with her heartburn, or it could be an autoimmune reaction. He recommended that she get a second opinion.

At the Mayo clinic, her doctor confirmed the diagnosis. He prescribed antacids along with Prednizone. "The antacids and medication helped a lot, but I knew that I wasn't really getting better," she says. "I still couldn't drive a car, balance my checkbook, or even concentrate enough to do needlepoint. My husband had to finish preparing dinner, do the dishes and all the laundry. I was still coughing constantly."

One thing Donna could do was read. After finishing a book on Maharishi Vedic Medicine, she turned to her husband and said, "I'm going to try this."

While in residence for five days at The Raj Maharishi Ayur-Veda Health Center in Fairfield, Iowa, she began Maharishi Rejuvenation therapy, which included oil massage, steam baths, and elimination therapy to clear away toxins and impurities. She also started a diet to reduce acid and heartburn, and took herbal supplements to bring her body back into balance. She learned special breathing techniques to strengthen her lungs, and the Transcendental Meditation technique to reduce stress and give her body the deep rest it needed to heal. After returning home, she continued a home-care program to decrease the cause of her disease and strengthen her body. She also continues to visit The Raj twice a year for Maharishi Rejuvenation treatments.

Today Donna no longer has to use Prednizone. She can hold an hour-long conversation without coughing. Her heartburn is gone, and she doesn't need antacids. Her blood pressure is normal, and her good cholesterol has doubled. On her last visit to The Raj, she drove herself and a friend the seven hours each way. Best of all, her contagious laugh is back.

At one point after starting Maharishi Rejuvenation treatments, Donna went to see her gastroenterologist. After examining her he said, "What are you doing?" She didn't know what he meant. "Let's put it this way," he said. "Most people in your situation don't get well. They only get worse. Whatever you're doing, just keep it up."

How *Maharishi Rejuvenation* Therapy Works

When Donna began Maharishi Rejuvenation therapy, she chose to be an inpatient. Whether you are an inpatient or an outpatient, your treatment starts with a diagnosis by a physician trained in Maharishi Vedic Medicine. The physician prescribes a program of treatments to address your specific needs. The treatments are administered by trained technicians and monitored by a medical doctor. Each of the therapies includes herbs chosen to balance and support your doshic constitution and treat your specific disorders. The treatments last anywhere from three to thirty days, and take from two to four hours each day. During the entire treatment the patient follows a special diet, which is light, warm, and easy to digest. This helps the body purify and eliminate ama.

The central feature of Maharishi Rejuvenation therapy is called *panchakarma. Pancha* means "five" and *karma* means "action." Panchakarma is the name for five special actions or procedures used to remove impurities from the body. It is a major part of the field of internal medicine known as *kayachikitsa,* which concerns sustaining and balancing the digestive fire (agni). Kayachikitsa also includes other procedures to purify and pacify the doshas, including *snehana* (internal purification to prepare for panchakarma), *swedana* (steam therapy), and *abhyanga* (oil massage). Maharishi Rejuvenation therapy includes all of these treatments, plus many others.

Snehana: Oleation Therapy

This first step of treatment is done at home for several consecutive days. The patient takes a small quantity of ghee (clarified butter) or a specific herbal tea to loosen, lubricate, and soften impurities. Cell walls have a lipid (fat) membrane that allows other fats and oils to pass through them. Ghee, being a fat, penetrates each cell of the body and loosens the impurities. (This includes the brain cells, because ghee can penetrate the blood-brain barrier.) This whole process is called oleation. Snehana is useful in treating dryness, anxiety, and urinary disorders.

Virechana: Laxative Therapy

Once the ghee or herbal tea has loosened cellular impurities, they are flushed out of the intestines with a mild laxative. To prepare for this treatment, the patient takes a warm bath. This dilates the channels of the body and helps loosened impurities flow from the peripheral areas through the circulatory system to the central area, the intestines. From there they are eliminated through the use of a mild laxative. Virechana is useful in skin and spleen disorders, diabetes, headaches, constipation, heart disease, asthma, coughs, gastrointestinal disorders, indigestion, and many other conditions.

Virechana is also one of the most powerful means to balance Pitta dosha, which is located in the stomach, liver, and pancreas. Virechana effectively gets rid of excess heat in any of these organs.

Massage Therapies

Abhyanga, Herbalized Sesame Oil Massage

This very enjoyable warm-oil, full-body massage is administered by two technicians who work simultaneously on both sides of your body, creating a balanced effect. The oil is specially treated with herbs that target the patient's particular imbalances. Skin, because of its porous nature, absorbs the herbalized oil like a sponge. This allows the healing herbs to reach the body tissues and loosen impurities and toxins at a very deep level.

Touch is a powerful sense—the only sense that is distributed over the whole body. Any touch is registered by the brain and affects the whole nervous system. During an abhyanga, the technicians work in synchrony on both sides of your head and body, so that the massage integrates the brain's left and right hemispheres and balances the whole body. Abhyanga balances Vata, the dosha associated with the sense of touch. Vata, as you will remember, leads the other doshas and is the main cause of physiological imbalance. So by balancing Vata, the abhyanga profoundly influences Pitta and Kapha as well. When you balance Vata, you can balance and settle your entire body.

Udvartana

This cooling massage treatment uses a paste made of ground grains. It cleanses the skin, increases circulation to the subcutaneous (deeper) tissues, and promotes weight loss.

Garshan

This massage uses wool or raw silk to increase circulation in the body. It helps eliminate clogging and impurities that might cause problems such as cellulite, and helps with weight problems.

Nasya

Nasya focuses on the head, neck, shoulders, and sinuses. In addition to massage, it involves two kinds of inhalation therapy—herbal drops to cleanse the nasal passages, and herbalized steam to clear mucus from the lungs and sinuses. Nasya stimulates the base of the brain and produces greater clarity and balance for the mind, brain, senses, and thyroid gland. Nasya was part of Donna's treatment, and it helped clear toxins from her chest, sinuses, and neck. It has beneficial applications for a stiff neck or jaw, tonsilitis, mouth diseases, facial palsy, headaches, goiter, earaches and lung diseases.

Fomentation (Heating) Treatments

Panchakarma uses different types of heat treatments. These dilate the srotas so that the impurities loosened through massage can be swept away. Heat also softens ama so that it is simpler to break down and eliminate. Once liquefied, ama enters the intestinal tract for easy evacuation. Heat treatments are prescribed for aches and pains in the joints, muscles, and bones—the accumulation sites for Vata and Kapha. They remove impurities throughout the musculoskeletal system.

Swedana

The patient is immersed in herbalized steam from the neck down. As a result, the sweat channels enlarge and impurities flow out. Swedana balances Vata and Kapha and benefits constipation, paralysis, asthma, and arthritis.

Pizzichilli

During this massage, the technicians continuously pour large quantities of warm oil all over the patient's body. The herbalized oil deeply penetrates the tissues, pacifies Vata, and eliminates any deep imbalances in the musculoskeletal system. Sometimes warm milk is substituted for oil, nourishing the skin as well as Vata dosha.

Pinda Swedana

Boluses, or cloth pouches filled with a mixture of herbs, rice, and milk, are massaged over the body. This technique adds nourishment, strength and balance to the joints and neuromuscular system.

Additional Treatments

Shirodhara

Warm oil is poured slowly back and forth across the forehead in a special pattern. The result is deep relaxation, brain-wave coherence and profound mental rest.

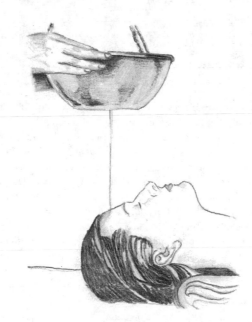

Netra Tarpina

The eyes are bathed in ghee and herbal smoke to help cleanse impurities and relieve any kind of eye strain.

Basti: Internal Cleansing Treatments

All of the heating and massage treatments above are designed

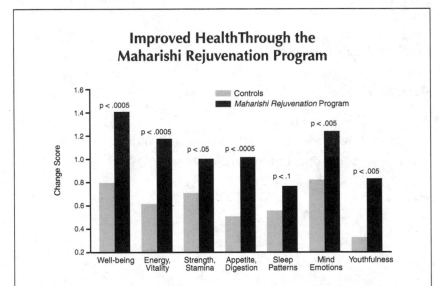

Improved HealthThrough the Maharishi Rejuvenation Program

This study compared 142 subjects who participated in a Maharishi Rejuvenation program for one week with 25 control subjects who received only intellectual knowledge of the program and its principles for the same amount of time. Changes in health symptoms were assessed with a health survey questionnaire. Those who received active treatment improved significantly in general well-being, energy and vitality, strength and stamina, appetite and digestive patterns, state of mind and emotions, and youthfulness and rejuvenation. They also reported improvement in previous health conditions. Control subjects did not show the same amount of improvement. This research indicates that, even after a short period of time, the Maharishi Rejuvenation program simultaneously improves many different areas of health. Other studies have found that this program also improves many aspects of mental health and cognitive performance. These findings support the hypothesis that the Maharishi Rejuvenation program promotes balance in both mind and body on a very fundamental level.

Reference: *The Journal of Social Behavior and Personality* vol, 5 (1990), pp. 1-27.

to dislodge impurities from the dhatus, organs, and srotas and allow them to flow into the intestinal tract. Bastis are internal cleansing treatments that flush out the intestinal tract with gentle oil and herbal enemas. This ensures that impurities leave the body quickly and safely.

Since the colon and lower pelvic area are the main seats of Vata, the basti is the most powerful treatment for balancing this dosha. This is actually the basti's primary purpose. Expelling impurities is its second objective.

Bastis fall into two categories, lubrication and elimination. The lubrication basti balances, nourishes, and strengthens the digestive tract, while the elimination basti causes thorough evacuation. Most treatment programs use both types and give them on alternate days.

The basti is considered a highly important therapy because it is exceptionally effective in normalizing Vata, the king of the doshas. Bastis are used for abdominal disease, constipation, loss of strength, diarrhea, chest pain, spleen disorders, fever, headache, earache, backache, tuberculosis, stiffness and many other Vata-induced disorders.

How *Maharishi Rejuvenation* Therapy Influences Health

Maharishi Rejuvenation therapy is one of the most potent therapies offered by Maharishi Vedic Medicine. It deeply transforms the body by removing impurities that prevent the body's inner intelligence from functioning properly. Although not everyone experiences as dramatic a shift in their health as Donna, patients consistently report greater energy, clarity of mind, well-being, and relief from a range of nagging health problems, from back pain to arthritis to acne.

Maharishi Rejuvenation therapy is highly esteemed in the Vedic tradition. The *Charaka Samhita* states, "The vitiated doshas alleviated by fasting and digestive herbs do at times get aggravated but those eliminated by elimination therapies do not recur. The doshas can be well compared with trees. Unless the tree is uprooted from its root, it will grow in spite of its branches, etc., being chopped off. Such is the case with the vitiated doshas. They go on causing diseases unless they are eliminated from their very root."[56]

The aim of Maharishi Rejuvenation therapy is to remove impurities before you get sick. Actually, your body constantly cleanses itself of impurities every moment you are alive. Your body not only regenerates millions of cells each week but also cleans up after itself. There is no comparison between your body's natural processes and man-made cleaning systems. It wouldn't be possible to devise a system as efficient as your body's waste disposal mechanisms. So panchakarma works simply to enhance your own, natural, internal cleansing processes.

The body's self-purifying operations—which include the kidneys, liver, bladder, bowels, skin, and lungs—work by collecting impurities and toxins and unloading them from the body. The problem is that over time, the body accumulates more toxins and wastes than it can effectively eliminate. When the wastes build up, they start to mask or block the body's governing intelligence. Disease develops and the body starts to age. For most modern-day people, free radicals and toxins are piling up faster than the body can dispel them. When impurities disrupt the work of the mind-body, a wide range of symptoms can arise, from fatigue, frequent colds, anxiety, and depression to serious disease.

Maharishi Rejuvenation therapy at the end of each season helps you start the next one in good health.

Supporting the Organizing Power of Consciousness

In addition to purification and doshic balance, rejuvenation treatments support the ability of consciousness, the body's governing intelligence, to do its job. The srotas form the infrastructure through which the physiological organizing power of consciousness flows.

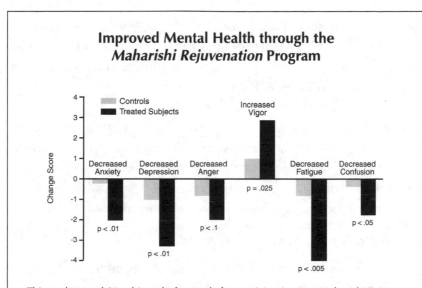

Improved Mental Health through the *Maharishi Rejuvenation* Program

This study tested 62 subjects before and after participating in a Maharishi Rejuvenation program for one week compared to 71 controls who received only intellectual knowledge of the program for the same amount of time. Changes in mental health were assessed by the Profile of Mood States, a standard psychometric instrument. The results showed statistically significant declines in unhealthy emotional states—anxiety, depression, fatigue, and confusion—and an increase in vigor.

These results indicate the Maharishi Rejuvenation program improves many aspects of the mind and emotions simultaneously. They demonstrate that a physical approach—the purification therapies of seasonal rejuvenation—can have a positive effect on mental health.

References: 1. Paper presented at the International College of Psychosomatic Medicine, Eighth World Congress, Chicago, Illinois, September 1985: Improvements in Health with the Maharishi Ayurveda Prevention Program.
2. *Journal of Social Behavior and Personality,* No. 5 (1990), pp. 1-27.

Blockage in the srotas diminishes or disrupts the essential operational influence of consciousness in every psychophysiological function.

Maharishi Rejuvenation therapy produces a massive wave of coherence, which sweeps away any obstructions in the srotas. When the srotas are clear, every mind-body system is guided by Natural Law.

As a computer programmer, Rolfe felt a lot of tension and

pressure on the job. Intense focus all day, every day, produced a spectrum of problems, including anger, worry, joint stiffness and gastrointestinal problems. Tall, thin, and blond, his physique and coloring revealed his Vata-Pitta doshic makeup.

Rolfe received Maharishi Rejuvenation treatments three times over the period of a year. His nervous stomach and stomach acid, as well as the stiffness in his muscles and joints, have disappeared. He described his experience, "The main thing I notice after panchakarma is more peace and relaxation, and also my body feels more light and frictionless, like a well-lubricated machine."

Herbalized Oils Treat Specific Imbalances

Maharishi Ayur-Veda Health Centers use special herbalized oils during Maharishi Rejuvenation therapy to treat specific disorders. These oils are meticulously prepared in India according to classical Ayurvedic methods. The process takes several days or even weeks and can involve as many as seventy-five different herbs. The herbal combinations are selected to target particular disorders and imbalances. Concentrated with herbs, the oils penetrate the skin and are metabolized by the whole body. They first remove ama from the skin. Then, by permeating the tissues, they remove blockages and ama from different subdoshas of Vata, Pitta, and Kapha.

Different oils are prepared for different panchakarma treatments, such as abhyanga, basti, and shirodhara.

In addition, specific herbalized ghees, called *ghritas*, provide a more precise and powerful way to purify the body before panchakarma, during the at-home preparation stage.

Not everyone receives the same oil for the same treatment. Body type and particular imbalances determine the oil for an individual's massage.

Two classes of oils are used, *saumya* and *tikshana*. Saumya oils remove physiological weakness. They gently address disease by purifying one dhatu after another. Tikshana oils penetrate and directly enter the body. They create heat in the blood, improved circulation, and purification. The oils soften the skin, gently seep into its pores, and allow healing herbs to mix directly with the blood. This process, called *vyavai vikasi*, eradicates blockages, dispels pain and heaviness, and inhibits the effects of pollutants to which the body is exposed.

Maharishi Ayur-Veda herbal compounds are also prescribed after panchakarma. These remedies match the oils used in the treatments. They resonate with the oils and magnify their beneficial effect.

Home Follow-Up Program

Chapter 17 described the value of giving yourself an abhyanga each morning at home, followed by a warm bath. The effect of self-massage is similar—though on a smaller scale—to the abhyanga you receive during Maharishi Rejuvenation therapy. It dislodges ama and opens the srotas. The hot bath dilates the srotas—arteries, veins, lymphatic channels, and so on—and the impurities then flow out, again, on a lesser scale, as they do during the heat treatments. This simple home routine helps maintain the results of Maharishi Rejuvenation therapy and prevents wastes and toxins from re-accumulating.

Rasayana Therapy

Once Maharishi Rejuvenation treatments have cleared the srotas, you are ready for rasayana therapy, the traditional herbal preparations that rejuvenate the mind-body and promote longevity. Medicinal herbs and rasayanas can have a much more powerful effect after panchakarma.

Together with rasayanas, the significant transformation that takes place through Maharishi Rejuvenation therapy has brought vitality and renewal to thousands of people. For the many individuals with chronic problems, they have brought an astounding resolution of what were once thought to be incurable illnesses.

CHAPTER 21

Restoring Wholeness with Sound and Other Natural Therapies

"The purpose of Maharishi's Vedic Approach to Health is to enliven the link between consciousness and matter—to create perfect health by maintaining lively co-ordination between the pure creative intelligence of Natural Law and its transformed values in the physiology."
—*Maharishi Mahesh Yogi*[57]

The therapies of Maharishi Vedic Medicine enliven the intelligence of Nature in the mind-body. In its unlimited, unmanifest state, Nature's intelligence is pure consciousness, pure awareness—a kind of infinite seed that contains the blueprint for the entire creation. All the impulses of intelligence and organizing power of Natural Law exist in consciousness in their unexpressed state—as pure potential—or what physics might describe as virtual activity in the unified field. Veda is pure consciousness, undivided wholeness, the nonmaterial totality of the impulses of Natural Law.

The abstract potential of Veda unfolds, or expresses itself, in a precise sequence. This Vedic process of manifestation is extraordinarily similar to the way that physics describes the emergence of creation from the unified field. The many Laws of Nature that organize and govern all physical processes in the universe originate from the abstract mathematical structures in the unified field.

Sound is the finest level of expression of the Veda. The sounds of the Veda unfold in a fixed sequence of syllables alternated with gaps of silence. These primordial sounds, in both their acoustic quality and their order of presentation, are the first and subtlest display of the Laws of Nature. They tell the complete story of the progressive unfoldment of the universe from its finest to its grossest forms. Consciousness, or the Veda, takes its first step toward becoming matter as sound, as patterns of vibration, and the entire creation consists of increasingly dense and complex manifestations of these fundamental vibrations.

Every part of the body, from microscopic DNA to large organs, and every physiological function, is an expression of the Veda, the omnipresent field of infinite knowledge and organizing power. Health depends on maintaining a lively connection between every element of the mind-body and the underlying blueprint in consciousness. If the organizing power of Nature's intelligence gets shadowed or blocked—or, we could say, if a part of the mind-body forgets how to function according to Nature's perfect design—the activity of that part of the body, and its wave pattern, get distorted. That element of the physiology then not only loses its individual capacity for healthy functioning, but also loses its connection to the governing intelligence of the mind-body as a whole. A break in the vibrational sequence for total psychophysiological health is created and disease results.

Vedic Sounds Create Orderliness

Listening to the Veda's primordial sounds can actually normalize the wave function in specific parts of the body or throughout the physiology.

The acoustic quality of specific sounds, syllables, and verses of the Vedic Literature embodies the pattern or blueprint for perfect form and function in corresponding areas of the mind-body. Any physiological weakness, any abnormal activity anywhere in the system, can be corrected by listening to or reading the associated aspect of the Veda and Vedic Literature. Maharishi Vedic Sound™ therapy helps the precisely correlated physiological elements remember how to function according to the original vibratory pattern embodied in that particular, sequential flow of impulses. For example, if the association fibers in the cerebral cortex have a problem, reading or listening to the part of the Veda that structures them—the *Yoga Sutras*—will help repair the damage. Just as the flow of a powerful river clears away any mud or deposits that block its natural course, the Vedic sounds help to remove physiological obstructions and aberrations, and to restore the original, perfect design of the human system. The value of these sounds does not lie in their musical quality—although they are pleasing to hear—but in their restructuring and ordering effect in the human system.

The Effects of Vedic Sounds on Cancer Cells

The last thirty years have brought a flood of research on the use of sound in healing. Today, music is used in oncology, surgery, anesthesiology, obstetrics, gerontology, and psychiatry. Researchers have found that music measurably affects the mind and body. Changes in the body's electrical conductivity, pulse rate, circulation, blood pressure, metabolism, internal secretions, muscular energy, respiratory rate, and oxygen consumption have all been reported. In general, soothing music lowers both oxygen consumption and basal metabolism, while exciting music creates more agitation in the body.[58]

Music has been found to reduce pain and decrease the necessity for pain medication by as much as 30 per cent.[59] In addition, multiple studies have shown that music can reduce the need for medication in a number of other conditions, such as severe headaches and painful neurological diseases.

At The Ohio State University College of Medicine, Dr. Hari

Sharma studied the effect of an area of the Veda called *Sama Veda* on human cancer. He found that the acoustic frequencies of Sama Veda decreased human cancer cell growth in vitro,[60] while hard rock music increased cancer cell growth in vitro. In his discussion of the research findings, Dr. Sharma noted that according to Maharishi Vedic Medicine, the primordial sounds of Sama Veda are the fundamental frequencies that form the human body and the entire universe. Listening to a traditional recitation of these sounds is predicted to have a rejuvenating and balancing effect on the body.

Although the exact mechanism for these findings needs to be investigated further, Dr. Sharma points out that modern physics sees all matter as a form of energy. Each type of matter pulsates in a certain frequency or wave pattern. For example, proteins and other macromolecules such as DNA are known to vibrate at low frequencies. In addition, cells have a certain vibration that reflects their function. If the cell becomes cancerous, the vibration changes.

Sama Veda is characterized by a slow, rhythmic, low-pitched, low-frequency sound. Dr. Sharma postulated that it may have strengthened the low-frequency vibrations of normal DNA, while inhibiting the growth of high-frequency cancer cells. Hard rock music, by contrast, involves many high-frequency tones and irregular rhythms, which may account for the fact that hard rock music generally increased the in vitro growth of cancer cells in the study. This research clearly shows that sound can have a powerful impact on the human physiology, and the consequent value of exposing the body and mind to life-supporting sounds. The Vedic syllables contain the same frequency patterns as the human body. They are therefore potentially the most effective acoustic tool for maintaining or restoring natural, orderly physiological activity.

Practical Applications

Two programs from Maharishi Vedic Medicine use Vedic sound to awaken the inner intelligence of the body. The Program for Chronic Disorders, described in Chapter 24, uses certain Vedic sounds to balance particular disorders. These may be used by patients in their daily lives over a long period of time.

A second regimen, Maharishi Vedic Vibration Technology^{SM}, provides virtually instant relief from a large number of both acute and chronic disorders. Patients receive an average of three 90-minute treatments for each disorder and frequently experience clear and positive results, either immediately or by the end of the series. During the treatments, trained practitioners select the sounds specific to each disorder, enliven the sounds in their own consciousness and then impart the sounds to the patients, using a subtle value of breath. The sounds reenliven the inner intelligence in diseased or dysfunctional areas of the mind-body, and the mental and physiological counterparts of that inner intelligence heal quickly.

Music Therapy

The melodies and rhythms of Maharishi Gandharva Veda^{SM} music reflect the natural rhythms of Nature and restore balance to the listener and the environment. The *ragas*, or musical patterns structured according to Vedic progressions of notes, are designed to be played at specific times of the day, according to a schedule in which each day is divided into twelve periods of two hours each.

Earlier you learned about the significance of Nature's cycles for your health. You know that different doshic qualities and Laws of Nature are lively at different times of the day and night. The morning air, for example, is fresh and alive—flowers open and birds sing—while in the evening, things settle down. To reflect these varying influences in Nature as the sun moves across the sky, specific ragas are played at the appropriate times. Each piece expresses the unique impulses of Nature that are lively during that period of the day or night, and brings the environment into harmony with those impulses.

Resisting the flow of natural cycles only causes strain. Maharishi Gandharva Veda music helps align your physiology with the impulses of Nature. In addition, it neutralizes atmospheric stress and creates peace in your home and society. It can be played in your home or office to create harmony and peace even when you are not there to hear it. It is also used in a clinical setting to balance the doshas and revitalize the mind and body.

Sound and Herbal Food Supplements

Just as everything in creation conveys a specific vibratory structure originating in the Vedic sounds, every herb carries a unique vibration. Herbs have a special connection with the human physiology. Each part of the body has the same vibratory impulse as a particular herb. In other words, the herb Maharishi Vedic Medicine prescribes for the lungs has the same frequency as a healthy lung. If a lung cell loses its connection with Nature's intelligence and therefore forgets how to operate normally, its wave or vibrational pattern becomes disturbed. The result is disease. The correct herb can restore the memory of healthy functioning to the diseased cell.

Herbs act like tuning forks, helping to reset the affected area in its natural frequency. The vibratory quality of the prescribed herb resonates with the part of the body that is diseased and restores the correct vibrational pattern. This is why herbs can directly influence precise areas of the body. They do not target disease, but instead resonate with the physiological component that has fallen out of sequence with the whole mind-body. When the wave pattern of the afflicted cells once again expresses its original vibrational blueprint and works in the proper sequence with the whole physiology, disease symptoms naturally disappear.

Aroma Therapy

Aroma therapy employs herb and flower extracts to diffuse healing scents into the air while you sleep. The herbs used in aroma therapy work much as they do in herbal formulas and are just as effective in restoring balanced functioning. Like the herbal compounds, Maharishi Vedic Medicine's aroma formulas use a combination of herb and flower essences which produce balance.

It's important to use the aroma oils in the traditional Vedic combinations. Otherwise, they could create an imbalance. For example, stimulating oils such as myrrh, juniper berry, and peppermint help normalize Kapha, which is responsible for weight gain and loss. However, individually any one of these oils could also create an unexpected Pitta imbalance, and could produce anger or ravenous hunger. This would be especially harmful for a person with a Pitta constitution or aggravated Pitta. The Maharishi Vedic Medicine aroma formula for weight loss takes care to offset this possibility by adding oils to soothe Pitta as well as Kapha. The result is an oil that stimulates weight loss without creating any imbalance.

Have you ever had the experience of smelling some delicious food cooking, such as bread or cookies, and found that the smell evoked a vivid memory of childhood? The sense of smell is particularly powerful because it is associated with the limbic area of the brain, which is linked with both emotions and memory. Consequently aroma therapy can help with a wide range of emotional as well as physical problems.

Ayurvedic pharmacology includes aroma formulas to balance each of the fifteen subdoshas. These are prescribed on the basis of a complete patient evaluation, including pulse diagnosis, to determine which subdoshas are out of balance. The aroma selection process is precise and individualized, and therefore a great deal more helpful than experimenting with aromatic oils from the health food store.

I have found these formulas to be extremely successful in correcting the underlying doshic imbalances at the root of disease. In addition, my patients tell me that they like this therapy because it is easy, inexpensive, and enjoyable. The herbal aromas are pleasing and soothing. They help repair your body and restore the memory of health effortlessly while you sleep.

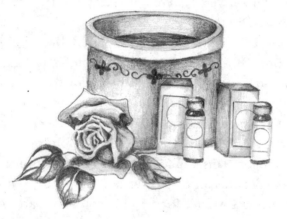

Healing through the Senses

You may have noticed that Maharishi Vedic Medicine includes all the senses. This chapter described techniques that use hearing (Maharishi Vedic Sound Therapy and Maharishi Gandharva Veda music therapy) and smell (aroma therapy). Earlier chapters discussed taste (diet and herbal supplements) and touch (abhyanga).

For most individuals, one or two of the senses are livelier or more awake, and this can be a function of their doshic constitution. People will often be particularly responsive to the therapeutic modality based on their strongest sense. Consequently, you may find that diet or herbal supplements are more effective than sound therapy, or vice versa. If you are predominately Kapha, you may have a strong sense of smell or taste, because those senses are related to earth and water, which are present in Kapha. If your constitution is dominated by Vata, you could be more sensitive to sound or touch, because they are related to air and space, the elements associated with Vata. Pitta can generate strong vision, because it corresponds to fire. In any case, using a variety of sensory therapies enlivens more sensory receptors in the body and creates a more holistic effect.

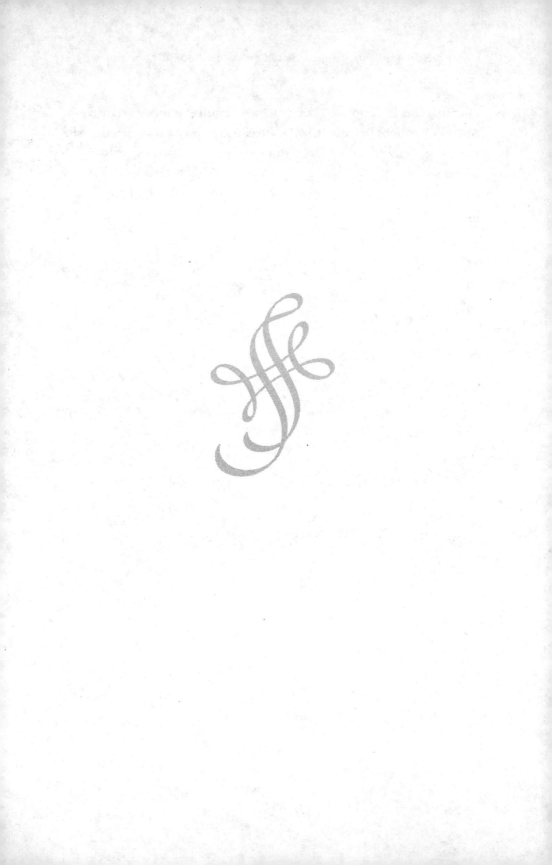

CHAPTER 22

Architecture in Accord with Natural Law

"Because the individual is cosmic, everything about individual life should be in full harmony with cosmic life. Maharishi Sthapatya Veda® design gives dimensions, formulas, and orientations to the buildings that will provide cosmic harmony and support to the individual for his peace, prosperity, and good health— daily life in accord with Natural Law, daily life in the evolutionary direction."   —*Maharishi Mahesh Yogi*[61]

The idea that home and work environments affect health is not new. People are increasingly aware that environmental toxins and pollutants have significant negative ramifications for health. Pesticides and chemicals have become suspected factors in a range of diseases. For example, the plastics, formaldehyde, and other chemicals in building materials have been implicated in "sick building syndrome," a general malaise characterized by fatigue and allergies. The Environmental Protection Agency estimates that thirty to seventy million U.S. workers are at risk of getting sick from the buildings in which they work—due to their construction materials, air quality, and so on. This amounts to a combined total of 150 million lost workdays, $59 billion in lost productivity, and $25 billion in medical bills each year.

Maharishi Sthapatya Veda design, one of the approaches of Maharishi Vedic Medicine, has addressed the need for life-supporting environments for several thousand years. This ancient science of Vedic architecture includes the modern ideal of nontoxic, natural building materials, but goes far beyond that. It also provides formulas for the design of buildings, towns, and cities that bring individual life into harmony with cosmic life. The aim of Maharishi Sthapatya Veda design is to help people live and work in buildings and communities that create health, happiness and prosperity.

Vastu

Many misfortunes and even diseases arise from lack of proper orientation of the structures in which people live and work, and from fundamental violations of Natural Law inherent in structural design. *Vastu*, a Sanskrit word that means "holistic structure of Natural Law," offers a detailed understanding of the relationship between a building, its site, and the local as well as distant environment—including the planets in the solar system. It incorporates such concepts as direction and placement. Each direction brings a particular influence, and Vedic architecture uses this knowledge to determine a structure's orientation as well as the placement of its rooms and furnishings. Vedic architecture factors in the topography, shape, size, and other characteristics of a building site to determine the best position for the building.

The ideal vastu, or building site, is selected to bring positive influences from the sun, moon, and planets. It defines the individual's connection to the universe and ensures that the activities performed within the home or office are in tune with the cosmos.

A model vastu is a square or rectangular shape within which a building is situated. It is aligned to the four main directions. In other words, its boundaries are true east-west and true north-south. A low wall should surround the boundaries of the vastu, and the property should have an east entrance. If there is any slope to the land, it should be to the north or east.

Correct Orientation

To create a perfect vastu, the Vedic architect must take into account three main principles: orientation, placement, and proportion. When a building design includes this knowledge, its inhabitants thrive. When it does not, inhabitants experience a cumulative strain and both health and finances may suffer.

Probably the most important influence on the vastu is its relationship to the movement of the sun. According to the Maharishi Sthapatya Veda program, the brain functions optimally when your house or office building faces east and the main door opens to the morning sun. The sun's energy is greatest when rising, and that power brings health and vitality to building occupants when the primary entrance looks east.

If a building faces north, this can also bring positive influences. However, when it faces any other direction (i.e., south, west, northeast, southeast, northwest, or southwest) a host of difficulties may result for health, finances, and professional or family life. Wrong orientation can even generate antisocial behavior. In Maharishi Sthapatya Veda architecture, a southern entrance is the most inauspicious. It blocks the support of Natural Law and brings negative influences to building residents or workers. Unfortunately, at least 75 per cent of all existing buildings have an inauspicious or unhealthy orientation.

If your body is not facing in the correct direction when you enter your home or perform a task, the brain's neurons do not function at their best. Biologists recently discovered that electrical activity in the thalamus changes according to the body's directional orientation. In addition, certain "place neurons" signal the brain when the body changes its orientation in a room or outdoor environment.

Maharishi Sthapatya Veda design not only lines up buildings in relationship to the rising sun, but also orients them with respect to the building lot's slope and shape, the location of bodies of water, road layout, and the surrounding environment. It also prescribes the right arrangement of furniture and appliances within the structure.

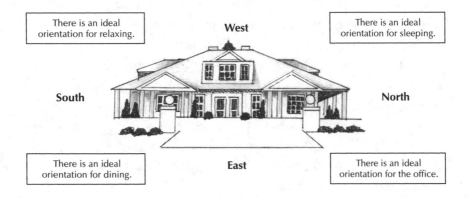

There is an ideal orientation for relaxing.	**West**	There is an ideal orientation for sleeping.
South		**North**
There is an ideal orientation for dining.	**East**	There is an ideal orientation for the office.

Correct Placement

Earlier in this book you learned how the sun's movement throughout the day and year creates powerful daily and seasonal cycles, which significantly affect health. Similarly, the sun's daily course through the sky affects activity within a building. As the sun shifts its position throughout the day, it radiates different qualities of energy that generate specific influences in different areas of a home. Consequently, each room needs to be placed where it will gain the maximum appropriate value of the sun's changing energy as it journeys across the sky.

The activity performed in every room should be supported by particular qualities of the sun's light and energy. For example, the kitchen needs the maximum sunlight to increase the energy for cooking food. Rooms used for sleeping and relaxing need less value of the sun. If a room is placed in the right spot, it will receive the best quality of solar energy for its function. The Maharishi Sthapatya Veda program describes the ideal location for entering, relaxing or entertaining, bathing, cooking, eating, sleeping, and conducting business.

Wrong room placements can confuse or strain building occupants and even cause health disorders. For example, you might feel sleepy in the study or hungry in the bedroom. If the kitchen is improperly situated, the food cooked there can create indigestion. If the bedroom is not in the right position, you could experience insomnia or chronic fatigue.

Correct Proportion

The size of the rooms in proportion to the entire home and the size of the home in proportion to the lot are also important. In Maharishi Sthapatya Veda architecture, the length and height of each wall, doorway, and window are calculated according to precise mathematical formulas, so that the proportions reflect underlying universal principles that align individual life with cosmic life.

When these three—orientation, placement, and proportion—are used to design not only life-supporting homes and workplaces but also entire communities, the quality of urban life can be significantly transformed. Imagine a community in which every element of the physical environment supports harmony in individual thinking and behavior with the laws that govern the entire universe. Imagine what it would mean if everyone experienced that connectedness. You could share in an unprecedented level of collective health and prosperity, and be free from every form of social disease, including war.

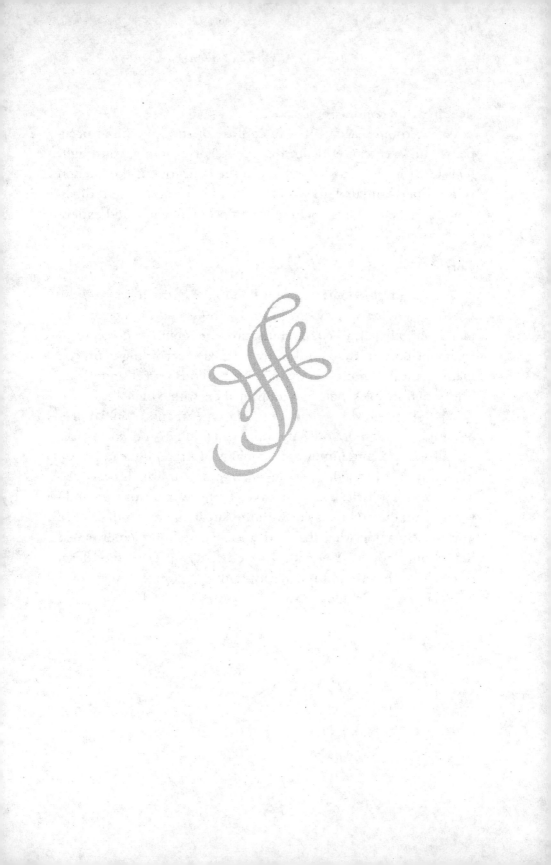

CHAPTER 23

Using Your Cosmic Connection to Create Health

"The centuries-old, medicine-predominant approach
to health has failed to eliminate sickness and suffering.
This is because medicine alone is too superficial to
influence all the innumerable values that constitute
the structure of life and its evolution. Only a holistic
approach that takes into consideration everything that
life is made of and everything that influences individual life, including the cosmic counterparts of the
physiology—sun, moon, and planets, etc.—can be
successful in handling health."

—*Maharishi Mahesh Yogi*[62]

You now have a basic picture of how your immediate environment—the buildings in which you spend your time—can affect
health. However, you are also strongly moved by the cosmic environment, the sun, moon and planets.

Most people know about the connection between the sun and
moon and the ocean's tides. The combined effect of the sun and
the moon generate the tides, although their primary cause is the
gravitational attraction of the moon. While this daily shift of billions of gallons of water is impressive enough, most people don't
realize that the Earth itself also experiences tides. The pull of the
sun and moon causes this planet to distort between about four
and one-half and fourteen inches each day. Interior lakes and
ponds do not appear to have tides because the water and the sur-

rounding land rise simultaneously.

When you consider what a powerful effect the moon and sun have on the Earth and its oceans, it is easier to grasp their effect on your own life. You are so intimately linked with the sun, moon, and planets in this solar system that you can think of them as your cosmic counterparts. One of the most fascinating approaches to Maharishi Vedic Medicine is the Maharishi Vedic Astrology℠ program, also called the Maharishi Jyotish℠ program. This precise mathematical system describes in detail the nature of this connection and its implications for individual life. It contains the science of transformation and the technology of prediction.

Determining Future Trends in Your Health

Some people are healthy all their lives and then suddenly hit a rough spot where everything seems to go wrong. Others struggle with one problem after another, despite their best efforts to maintain their health. Most often, people do not fully understand why these crises occur. They may feel like victims of a capricious universe, or they may wonder if the situation could have been prevented with adequate foreknowledge.

A Maharishi Vedic Astrology consultation explains the events and circumstances of individual life and their timing in terms of planetary cycles. It can do so because: (1) Everything in the universe, from the smallest particle to the largest star or planet, emerges from and is governed by that same infinite organizing power of pure consciousness; and (2) Evolution is an orderly process. Acorns become oak trees, not gardenias, and that growth process is precise and predictable. The entire creation, including each human life, emerges from the unified field in an exact sequence, not unlike a production line. If you know the sequence of steps involved in the production of a particular item, you can look at that item at any point in its development and know which steps have been completed and which remain.

An expert in the Maharishi Vedic Astrology program understands the Laws of Nature associated with planetary influences and human evolution, and can look at the pattern of any individual life and compute which events have already occurred and which ones are still on the way. Every aspect of life, including health, is understood in the context of the whole picture of an individual's life and growth, and every event can be known in advance.

The Maharishi Vedic Astrology program can alert you to any future trends, whether good or bad, in all areas of your life, including finances, family, profession, or health. It can also identify any specific periods that might need extra attention. If an accident or sickness looks likely, information can be given about remedial measures that can be used to avoid or minimize the difficulty.

Basic Principles of Prediction

Maharishi Vedic Astrology program experts calculate an individual birth chart, which is an orderly mathematical expression of the universe at the time of birth. It's like a snapshot of all the cosmic influences at play at that moment, and it provides a time-governed map of your journey through life. It includes all the information about the starting point and where you are going. The charts use three basic elements: nine *grahas* (planets), twelve *rashis* (signs or constellations), and twelve *bhavas* (houses, or fields of experience). Each rashi is composed of two or more clusters of stars, called *nakshatras*, which provide an additional influence on the individual.

The Nine Grahas (Planets)

Abbreviation	Sanskrit Name	English Name
Sy	*Surya*	Sun
Ch	*Chandra*	Moon
Ma	*Mangala*	Mars
Bu	*Budha*	Mercury
Gu	*Guru*	Jupiter
Sk	*Shukra*	Venus
Sa	*Shani*	Saturn
Rh	*Rahu*	Ascending lunar node*
Kt	*Ketu*	Descending lunar node*

The Twelve Rashis (Constellations)

Number	Sanskrit Name	English Name
1	*Mesha*	Aries
2	*Vrishabha*	Taurus
3	*Mithuna*	Gemini
4	*Karka*	Cancer
5	*Sinha*	Leo
6	*Kanya*	Virgo
7	*Tula*	Libra
8	*Vrishchika*	Scorpio
9	*Dhanu*	Sagittarius
10	*Makara*	Capricorn
11	*Kumbha*	Aquarius
12	*Meena*	Pisces

*The two lunar nodes are the points in space where the moon's path appears to intersect the sun's path, as viewed from the Earth.

Janma Kundali: the Birth Horoscope

The basic tool used in the Maharishi Vedic Astrology program is the birth horoscope, or *janma kundali,* which shows the positions and relationships of the grahas, rashis, bhavas and nakshatras at the time of birth.

To cast a birth horoscope, the person's time, date, and place of birth is used. Here is an example of a janma kyudali chart:

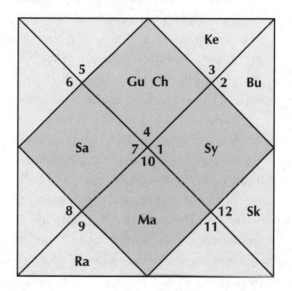

The janma kundali is divided into twelve squares to represent the twelve rashis and bhavas. Each number in the chart corresponds to the rashi in the previous list. The abbreviations match those in the list of grahas.

The Cosmic Counterparts

The Maharishi Vedic Astrology program scientifically describes the link between different aspects of your body and the planets of the solar system. Dr. Tony Nader, introduced in Chapter 3, discovered that the different aspects of human physiology form an exact replica of the patterns of intelligence contained in the Veda and Vedic Literature. In that context, he also found a one-to-one correlation between Jyotish—one of the forty aspects of Vedic Literature—and the basal ganglia. When you look at a cross-section of the brain, this correspondence is quite clear. The thalamus—the largest and most central of the basal ganglia—parallels the sun; the hypothalamus, the moon; the amygdala, or red nucleus, Mars; the subthlalamus, Mercury; globus pallidus, Jupiter; substancia nigra, Venus; and putamen, Saturn.

The function of each planet, as defined by the Maharishi Vedic Astrology program, parallels the function of each of the brain's basal ganglia. For example, the thalamus, which reflects the role of the sun, occupies a central place in the brain, and all the basal ganglia and sensory and motor inputs connect to it. This correspondence graphically illustrates the fundamental intimacy between microcosm as expressed in the human physiology and macrocosm—the total created universe.

The evolution of the universe and its endless variety of individual components is administered by Natural Law. The Maharishi Jyotish program takes the Vedic knowledge of the Laws of Nature, which structure the sequential expression of every element of creation, and applies them to the events and conditions of human life. It demonstrates that deep link between individual life and the vast web of Nature of which you are a part—so deep a link that the planets really are the cosmic counterparts of the ingredients of your life.

Averting Future Health Problems

The Vedic Literature advises, "Avert the danger that has not yet come." The Maharishi Vedic Astrology program is a practical science. If you find out that an accident or health problem lies in the future, you can take steps to avoid it. You can consult a physician and begin to take preventive measures to ensure good health

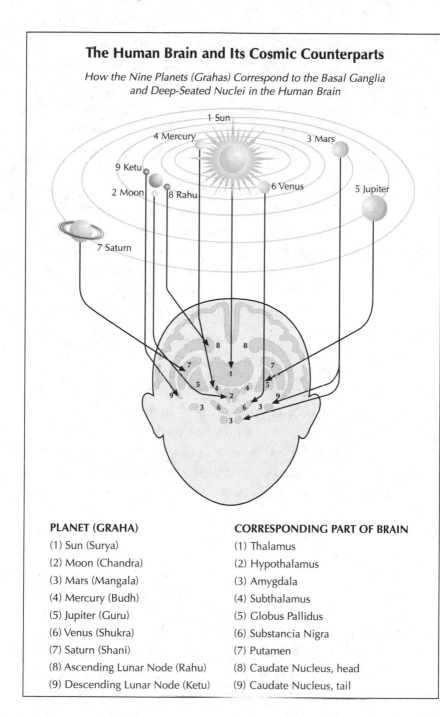

The Human Brain and Its Cosmic Counterparts

*How the Nine Planets (Grahas) Correspond to the Basal Ganglia
and Deep-Seated Nuclei in the Human Brain*

PLANET (GRAHA)	CORRESPONDING PART OF BRAIN
(1) Sun (Surya)	(1) Thalamus
(2) Moon (Chandra)	(2) Hypothalamus
(3) Mars (Mangala)	(3) Amygdala
(4) Mercury (Budh)	(4) Subthalamus
(5) Jupiter (Guru)	(5) Globus Pallidus
(6) Venus (Shukra)	(6) Substancia Nigra
(7) Saturn (Shani)	(7) Putamen
(8) Ascending Lunar Node (Rahu)	(8) Caudate Nucleus, head
(9) Descending Lunar Node (Ketu)	(9) Caudate Nucleus, tail

and dissolve any imbalance that might lead to disease.

In some cases, the Maharishi Jyotish program consultant (*pandit*) will prescribe a *yagya*, a procedure to neutralize the planetary energies that have already led to ill health or may do so in the future. Maharishi Yagya performances are precise Vedic procedures conducted by Vedic pandits in India who are thoroughly trained in this ancient knowledge.

While Maharishi Yagya performances can assist in any area of life—such as marriage, home, children, or financial success—one of their most important uses is to avoid illness or accidents. A Maharishi Vedic Astrology program consultant can identify planetary trends in your life that hold the potential for disease or may have already generated it. He can then recommend Maharishi Yagya performances to counteract these negative influences and support any medical treatments.

How *Maharishi Yagya* Performances Work

Maharishi Yagya performances generate specific life-supporting influences that counteract detrimental effects and enhance beneficial ones. To understand how this works, think of the principle of action and reaction. When you throw a stone in the water, it creates waves that reach the shore and eventually return back to you. Similarly, your thoughts and actions engender influences that reverberate throughout the universe. Every thought, feeling, and action has an effect—whether positive or negative—that will return to you in time.

The birth chart tells how and when that returning influence will affect you. If the influence is negative, and the individual faces a period of weak health or family problems, for example, the Maharishi Jyotish program expert will recommend a Maharishi Yagya performance to dissipate the impact of the adverse planetary pattern at its root. Other times yagyas are prescribed to enhance a good period, so that the individual enjoys the full potential of the favorable trends. In both cases, the Maharishi Yagya performance produces a flood of harmonious, constructive influences.

Effective Performance

The most important requirement for a successful yagya is that it be conducted from the level of pure consciousness. Maharishi Yagya performances are conducted in India by Maharishi Vedic pandits who have been meticulously trained under the guidance of Maharishi Mahesh Yogi. The pandits have been deeply grounded in the Vedic tradition, and they carry out the ceremonies from the deepest level of their awareness. This unique training and procedure ensures that the yagya has the full effect predicted by the Vedic texts.

**Applying the *Maharishi Jyotish* Program and
the *Maharishi Yagya* Program to the Treatment of Disease**

The Maharishi Jyotish and Maharishi Yagya programs provide unique tools for diagnosis and treatment that are not available in Western medicine. As pointed out earlier, the successful treatment of illness lies in the ability to correctly diagnose and eliminate its root cause. If a person is already sick, the Maharishi Jyotish program identifies the cosmic elements that have led to this condition. This precise analysis of the birth chart is an invaluable diagnostic procedure, because it defines the exact nature and primary source of the disease.

Once the nature and basis of disease are ascertained, the Maharishi Yagya program can be used as a remedial measure to help counteract the causal factors and support medical treatments. However, Maharishi Vedic Astrology consultations also describe future pathogenic patterns. This makes it possible to have the yagyas performed before the manifestation of illness, which can minimize it or even eliminate it entirely. Maharishi Yagya performances are most effective when they are done before events or symptoms actually arise.

It is important to recognize that these technologies are only supplements to standard medical treatment. They support diagnosis and treatment and should never be used as a substitute. Maharishi Vedic Medicine includes many approaches and each one has its particular value for the successful treatment of chronic disease.

For example, a 35-year-old woman was diagnosed with rheumatism, an autoimmune disease. At the onset she suffered from joint stiffness, trouble with circulation, deterioration of the muscles, and weakening of vital organs. Blood tests showed that antibodies were attacking the muscles around her heart, and her doctor prescribed high doses of Prednizone to prevent heart problems. The Prednizone had its own side effects: swelling in her face, mood swings, anger, and a sense of being emotionally and physically out of balance.

She reported, "By practicing various approaches of Maharishi Vedic Medicine [Maharishi Rejuvenation therapy; Maharishi Ayur-Veda herbal supplements, diet and daily routine; the Transcendental Meditation and TM-Sidhi programs] my symptoms lessened and then disappeared. I was able to discontinue the use of Prednizone altogether."

Then the disease flared up again. She was told that she would have to return to high doses of Prednizone, which she was reluctant to do because of the negative side effects.

"I decided to do the Maharishi Yagya program," she said. "The very first morning I noticed immediate results. My body felt so much lighter, balanced, and integrated. From there my health turned around and started improving each day. The Maharishi Yagya performances stopped the symptoms and I did not have to take the Prednizone after all, which was a huge relief."

Another patient noted, "Six months after the Maharishi Yagya performance, my health is much better and the likelihood of further cardiac infarction has become remote. I feel more stable and confident."

Some people find that the yagyas influence their mental health, as this man described. "It has been many months since the Maharishi Yagya performances, and I continue to feel really great. My fears and phobias are disappearing, one after the other. I am very satisfied."

Health is a state of perfect integration of mind and body. When the body and mind are functioning at their best, they replicate the structure of the Veda, the fundamental totality of Natural Law. Every element of the mind-body—from DNA to cells, to organs and limbs—functions perfectly within itself and with the whole system. Moreover, individual physiology works in complete harmony with cosmic physiology, the body of the universe. The Maharishi Yagya program, like all the aspects of Maharishi Vedic Medicine, helps you align yourself with Natural Law and experience the full integration of microcosm (your own physiology) with macrocosm (the entire universe).

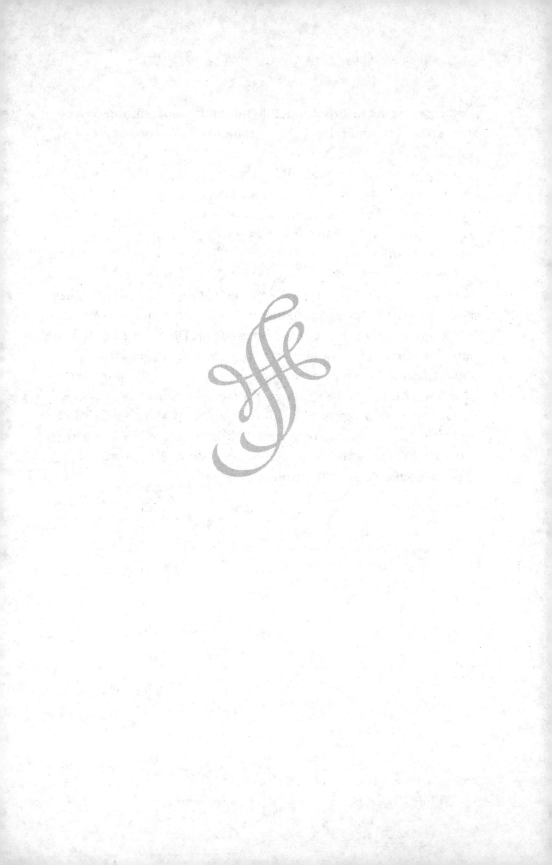

CHAPTER 24

In-Residence Programs for Profound Healing

"Veda is the common inner intelligence of everyone's body. People have not known it, and this ignorance of one's own inner healthy intelligence is the cause of all the difficulties of the physiology, and all disease. So my message for every individual is to have this knowledge of the inner intelligence of the body, and on this basis live perfection in life." —*Maharishi Mahesh Yogi*[63]

Many patients find it difficult to continue their daily lives while trying to recover from a chronic disease. In many cases, they need in-residence care. This is certainly ideal, as the patient can then rest fully, stay focused on healing, and take part in intensive treatment programs. The recovery from chronic disease in these cases is often much faster.

Two classes of Maharishi Rejuvenation therapy (panchakarma) are available, in-residence and outpatient. In outpatient panchakarma, the participant lives at home and continues his or her job, while spending a few hours a day receiving treatment. Though not as restful, it is still extremely effective, and more convenient for people who have family and work responsibilities and who want seasonal panchakarma on a regular basis. The majority of panchakarma treatments in the United States have been given in an outpatient setting at local Maharishi Vedic Medicine clinics.

In-residence panchakarma allows people to come to a secluded environment, protected from the demands of normal life, where food and personal needs are taken care of. The classical Ayurvedic texts recommend this for a more profound purification experience. Maharishi Ayur-Veda Health Centers and the Centers for Chronic Disorders offer restful, comfortable environments, where people can forget their normal responsibilities and experience profound physiological transformation.

These centers* specialize in intensive care and offer the most comprehensive Maharishi Vedic Medicine programs available for treatment of chronic disorders. Their programs were developed under the direction of an international panel of experts in Maharishi Vedic Medicine, and use all forty aspects of the Maharishi Vedic Approach to Health. New therapeutic elements include the ways in which treatments are applied and combined, powerful levels of treatment, and special herbs and techniques that are not available elsewhere. The therapeutic regimens at the Maharishi Ayur-Veda Health Centers and the Centers for Chronic Disorders are available in various formats for various lengths of stay. The Chronic Disorder Program, which is available in most of these centers, generally consists of three weeks of concentrated, in-residence care. It includes:

- A comprehensive patient evaluation
- A personalized treatment program designed and supervised by a specially trained physician
- Individualized diet and daily routine
- Specific herbal food supplements
- Maharishi Rejuvenation (panchakarma) treatments
- Therapies to balance the near environment (the Maharishi Sthapatya Veda program)
- Therapies to balance the distant environment (the Maharishi Vedic Astrology and Maharishi Yagya programs)

---

*At the time of this writing, there are five such centers in the United States and three in Canada (see Appendix).

- Maharishi Vedic Sound therapy
- Additional therapies from the Maharishi Vedic Approach to Health as needed
- Highly personalized care throughout the day
- A home treatment program

The results have been impressive. Take, for example, a patient we'll call Andrea. Andrea had suffered from Parkinson's disease for eleven years before she came to the Center for Chronic Disorders in Dallas, Texas. When she arrived, she had trouble walking, due to severe side effects from the allopathic medicine she was taking.

"The results were more significant than anything I have ever tried," she said. "Because of the side effects from my Western medicine, my legs were so spastic I couldn't walk. I was constantly losing my balance, and I felt a pressure on my eyes so bad I couldn't even touch them. All of that is completely gone. Overall my symptoms improved about 40 to 50 per cent, and I was able to reduce my medicine to half, something that is pretty much unheard of for people with Parkinson's disease."

Another patient, Sonia, was sick for only one year before she sought out the Center for Chronic Disorders, but her problems were equally drastic. She had developed a tumor the size of a small orange on her right elbow, and another tumor under her foot kept her from walking normally. Tumors in her lungs made her breathing labored and an inflammation irritated her eyes. She felt depressed and was immobilized by overall achiness and flu-like symptoms.

A battery of tests and visits to specialists diagnosed her problems as a type of gout, iritis, and rheumatism. Doctors prescribed five different medicines to relieve the pain and halt the development of the tumors, but they did not help much. Finally, she visited the Ochsner clinic in New Orleans. There she was told that all her symptoms were due to a rare immune system disorder called sarcoidosis. Although relieved to finally have a correct diagnosis, Sonia was dismayed to find that no known treatment for her disease existed.

At this point Sonia decided to enroll in the three-week, in-residence treatment program at the Center for Chronic Disorders in Dallas. She found almost immediate relief. "At first, I would go in for my treatments each morning aching and full of pain, almost unable to get up on the treatment table," recalled Sonia. "Afterward I felt tremendous. Every day this happened. Then I just started feeling better continuously. At that point, my symptoms started to drop off one by one, and to my relief, the tumors started to shrink."

After returning home, Sonia carefully followed the home treatment program prescribed by her doctors. The tumor on her elbow and her lung problems disappeared, and her eye inflammation improved. "The effects really are like night and day," Sonia reported. "Before, I had all these terrible problems, and now I just don't have them anymore. It was just remarkable. I could be dead if I hadn't had the opportunity to do this."[64]

Diseases Treated by the Chronic Disorder Program

- Coronary heart, kidney, and liver disease
- Chronic fatigue
- Hypertension
- Benign prostatic hyperplasia
- Chronic bronchitis and bronchial asthma
- Weight problems
- Gallstones
- Psoriasis
- Chronic sinusitis, headaches, and back pain
- Hyperacidity
- Eczema
- Peptic ulcer

- Rheumatoid arthritis and osteoarthritis
- Irritable bowel syndrome and inflammatory bowel disease
- Hypothyroidism and hyperthyroidism
- Menstrual problems and menopausal syndrome
- Diabetes (non-insulin dependent)
- Alzheimer's, connective tissue, and Parkinson's disease
- Depression and chronic anxiety
- Multiple sclerosis

The luxurious Maharishi Ayur-Veda Health Centers in Fairfield, Iowa, (The Raj) and Lancaster, Massachusetts, also offer prevention programs for healthy people who want to bolster their immunity and neutralize imbalances before they develop into disease. Besides Maharishi Rejuvenation therapy, two of their most potent therapeutic regimes are the Veda-Intensive Program for Chronic Disease and the Maharishi Rasayana Program^{SM}.

The Veda-Intensive Program for Chronic Disease

Structured especially for people with chronic disease, this program is offered in residence for three-, four-, or five-week options. It includes purification treatments similar to Maharishi Rejuvenation therapy, but the treatments are much deeper and tailored for specific conditions. The patient also receives a personalized diet and disease-specific rasayanas, powerful herbal healing agents to purify and nourish the mind and body and eliminate disease.

Maharishi Rasayana Program

This is the most advanced level of health enhancement for those who are already healthy. Given in residence, the patient receives powerful, penetrating Maharishi Rejuvenation treatments while taking special rasayanas. This treatment can last ten, twenty, or thirty days, and brings a profound level of rejuvenation and physiological refinement.

These comprehensive in-residence programs for chronic disease can create a new era in which chronic disease is both treatable and rare, so that you can enjoy a life that is not only free of pain and physiological restriction, but also full of vitality and happiness.

CHAPTER 25

Beyond Medicine:
A Vision of the Future

"In order to bring about the transformation of anything into anything, the intelligence of the scientist
must operate from the transcendental level, which is
the basic level of intelligence of every object in creation.

"Functioning from transcendental, self-referral intelligence, any individual can accomplish anything in the
whole field of creation—in the whole field of the ever-
expanding universe."   —*Maharishi Mahesh Yogi*[65]

It is difficult to fathom how brilliantly the universe is administered. Its size alone challenges the imagination. Consider this:
The nearest star system is the Centauri system, a group of three
stars which is 4.4 light years away—a distance of over one billion
trips around the Earth. It would take thousands of years for one
of our spaceships to reach it. The nearest galaxies are even far-
ther away. Each galaxy is composed of one million to one trillion
stars, held together by their gravitational pull. Our own galaxy,
the Milky Way, is part of a local group of galaxies—the ones clos-
est to us in the Milky Way. This local group includes at least
twenty-seven galaxies and covers an area approximately three million light-years in diameter. The universe is filled with an un-
countable number of such galaxy groups.

The managing intelligence in the human body is equally fan-
tastic. The human body mirrors the inconceivable variety and

complexity of the cosmos. For example, your genetic code is found in each cell in your body in the form of DNA. If you've ever seen a replica of DNA, you can't help but marvel at the intricacy, delicacy, and beauty of its design. Like a carefully crafted piece of jewelry, DNA spirals in a long coil called a double helix. Incredibly, the tiny DNA molecule, composed of twenty-three gene pairs and various amino acids, contains the intelligence necessary to form and flawlessly govern all the cells of the human mind and body, including 100 billion neurons in the brain and 100 trillion cells in the body.

After hundreds of years of modern science, we have only begun to understand this miracle. The nature of the intelligence which orchestrates this immense and complex universe is unfathomable. The intelligence and organizing power of DNA is equally amazing. In fact, they are one and the same.

The Human Physiology Is Cosmic

The Laws of Nature that govern the swinging of your arm also govern the planets swinging through space. Your body and all life—from the smallest particle to the most immense galaxy—are expressions of the same abstract field of pure consciousness. It is a field of unlimited possibilities. The blueprint for everything the universe can become is there in the state of pure potential, the total potential of Natural Law. The Veda is this unified state of the nonmaterial fabric of Natural Law. Your mind and body manifest the perfect orderliness of the Veda in every structure and function, and DNA contains the musical scores for the entire repertoire of the miraculous human symphony.

What significance does this knowledge have for health? If every human being is an expression of the Veda, then everyone also embodies the total potential of Natural Law. That means the same vast intelligence, creativity, and organizing power that runs the entire cosmos is within each and every person. If you fully realized this potential, your life could become a continuum of unlimited joy and success. This is what you are designed to experience. The elimination of pain and disease is just one benefit, just a beginning. Your life can flow with the same perfection, momentum, expansiveness, and brilliance of a trillion galaxies whirling through space. Medicine as we know it would then be obsolete.

Your Vedic Physiology

Professor Tony Nader, M.D., Ph.D., made a striking medical breakthrough several years ago, which was introduced in Chapter 2. He had been working intensively with Maharishi for many years, exploring the correspondences between the Vedic paradigm and the Western medical tradition. Essentially, Dr. Nader discovered Veda and Vedic Literature in the human physiology. That is, he located exact correlations between physiological structures and functions and particular aspects of the Veda. You could say that every part of your mind body is a precise expression of some aspect of the Veda and Vedic Literature. And the intelligence within your physiology and brain is the same as the structure of the Veda and Vedic Literature within the field of pure consciousness, the Unified Field of Natural Law.

In his book *Human Physiology—Expression of Veda and the Vedic Literature*[66], Dr. Nader offers a comprehensive picture of the connections between the Veda and every facet of human form and function. For example, he points out that Nyaya, an area of the Vedic Literature that describes the qualities of intelligence responsible for distinguishing and deciding, has the thalamus as its physiological counterpart. Nyaya even provides a clear and thorough depiction of the structure and function of the thalamus.

Dr. Nader's book also delineates the correspondence between the parts of our brain and the solar system. The thalamus, which occupies the center of the brain, corresponds to the sun. The moon correlates with the hypothalamus, Mars with the amygdala,

Mercury with the subthalamus, Jupiter with the globus pallidus, Saturn with the putamen, and Venus with the substancia negra.

Each individual is constructed according to the same blueprint as the immediate physical universe and, ultimately, the entire cosmos.[67] Each person on earth expresses the same, unbounded intelligence of Natural Law that permeates the cosmos in his or her own physiological structure and functioning.

Unfolding the Full Potential of Life

While each individual has the same enormous capacity for health, achievement, and fulfillment, clearly some people are using more of it than others. Some people are healthy and full of energy and enthusiasm, while others feel tired and defeated or sick. Some people are able to think clearly and achieve their objectives with relative ease, while others struggle or fail. Are some people born with intelligence and good health, while others are not? Or are some people healthy and successful because they live in a way that maximizes their potential?

Recent research shows that any kind of sensory or emotional experience leaves a trail in the structure of the brain. If the stimulus is repeated often enough, the neurons take a certain shape, forging a connection we call memory. If the brain lacks a nourishing stimulus, the affected neurons die. This means that certain necessary connections for physiological functioning are lost. Depending on individual experience, especially in the early years, some neurons perish while others flourish, creating a set neuronal pattern. Only part of the brain is used, while its holistic functioning—including the tiny connections among trillions of neurons—may be lost.

Modern education helps reinforce limited development of the brain's potential. If a student is trained to be a mathematician, a specific part of the brain is activated. If the student is trained to be a musician, another part is stimulated. When modern education channels students into specialized fields where only small portions of the brain are used, many neuronal connections are lost and, along with them, the brain's natural capacity for holistic functioning. What is needed is an educational program that wakes up the full capacity of the brain.

Listening to or reading the Vedic Literature does just that. It helps to restore the missing connections between neurons and to reconstruct the brain's holistic potential. If you expose the mind-body to the primordial frequencies of the Veda, you experience the full value of Nature's managing intelligence in every aspect of brain function.

A recent pilot study demonstrated how the Vedic sounds develop the whole brain. Fred Travis, Ph.D., and other researchers at Maharishi University of Management in Fairfield, Iowa, found that reading the Vedic Literature in Sanskrit (the language of the Veda) created a state of heightened awareness, marked by increased brain wave coherence. The EEG patterns were similar to those that appear during the practice of the Transcendental Meditation technique. When study participants read French, English, or Spanish, their EEG patterns did not display the same increased coherence. Reading modern languages involved only a localized area of the brain, whereas reading the Vedic Literature in Sanskrit increased orderliness in the brain as a whole.

At birth, everyone contains the flawless structure of Veda in his or her own consciousness, but it must be fully enlivened. All of the programs of Maharishi Vedic Medicine described in this book aim to awaken the dynamic flow of consciousness in every aspect of life.

How the Inner Intelligence of the Body Can Eliminate Pain

In a chronic disease such as asthma, certain neurons and cells have stopped operating normally and are no longer fully connected to the organizing power of Nature that administers the many complex functions of the human physiology. Once one part of the body stops working properly, other parts may react or try to compensate and can also be thrown out of gear. In the case of asthma, some cells start to constrict, while others start to produce excess fluid. The net result is that the individual with asthma has trouble breathing and experiences pain, panic, and anxiety.

If the neurons and cells can distort or become disorderly, they can also recover. They can stop reacting—producing excess fluid, tension, spasms—in a second.

For example, if you can move your hand one way, you can move it back. Let's say your hand is extended, all five fingers stretched out. To make a fist, some muscle cells have to relax; others have to tense. The speed of these motions has to be calculated and the nerve endings have to send thousands of messages. It would take a week to calculate and describe what it takes to shift from an open hand to a tight fist. If you analyzed the problem piecemeal, it would seem impossible to do in one second's time. Yet your body naturally makes such movements all day long, most of which you take for granted.

This same naturalness characterizes the phenomenon of Maharishi Vedic Vibration Technology. When your physiology receives gentle impulses of orderliness in the form of Vedic sounds, it automatically shifts back to its healthy pattern of functioning, aligned with Nature's intelligence. The mind-body's managing intelligence organizes the movement of a hand simply and automatically. With equal simplicity, physiological disorder can be transformed into order.

Practical Applications of Maharishi Vedic Medicine to Relieve Pain

The idea of "instant relief" may sound like science fiction to many people, but since the Maharishi Vedic Vibration Technology's inception in 1997, research and subjective testimony have repeatedly confirmed its reality. In the first study, done in November 1997 in Berlin, more than 400 patients from Holland, Germany, and France received Maharishi Vedic Vibration Technology consultations. Eighty per cent of the patients reported good or very good results. Pain and discomfort decreased after just a few minutes. This was true even in cases of long-standing, seemingly intractable problems. Patients experienced relief from back problems, arthritis, headache, asthma, insomnia, psoriasis, and many other complaints.

An American physician, Dr. Edwards Smith, specialist in internal medicine and rheumatology and a Fellow of the American College of Physicians, was a member of the team of research scientists who witnessed several patients' remarkable recoveries. He reported, "A jurist suffering from tennis elbow [an arthritic condition] was unable to lift a chair before the treatment. Immediately afterwards he lifted it high in the air five consecutive times by holding one leg of the chair with the previously injured arm. This is how he was trying to convince himself of his recovery, but he was cautioned by the experts that he should avoid such undue strain while that part of the body was still in the process of recovering its normal functioning.

"On two different occasions I watched two ladies enter the room very slowly. Each step was obviously painful. One was using two crutches. The other was using two canes. Both had been suffering for over thirty years from severe arthritic problems in the lower extremities. I saw each of them come out of the room after a few minutes of treatment. They were walking almost normally, without crutches or canes. In her effort to try out her ability to walk without pain, one of them seemed to be dancing with a smile of surprise. It was the fulfillment of my career as a doctor to see this."

One patient had suffered from migraine headaches for fifteen years, and from asthma since the age of eight. Before the treatment she was short of breath and had headaches. Afterward she reported that her chest felt free and light. She had no more head pain and she had an overall feeling of light and freshness. A patient who had suffered from arthritis since 1984 said that the pain in his bones as well as his headaches had disappeared.

In 1999, more than 2,000 people in the United States received Maharishi Vedic Vibration Technology consultations. Their self-evaluations are currently being analyzed. Initial findings show an average improvement of 42.3 per cent. This is quite remarkable when it's taken into account that the conditions being addressed were largely chronic, with an average duration of 13.8 years, and that the relief was usually gained within four or five days. The conditions being treated included a full range of mental as well as physical problems. The results for anger, depression, anxiety, emotional instability, and grief showed an average improvement of 50.6 per cent.

Many doctors now feel both amazed and grateful as they see patients with seemingly intractable problems improve. Dr. Nancy Lonsdorf in Washington, D.C., reports that a patient who had suffered from eczema-related itching since childhood had nearly normal skin within two weeks after his treatment. A man recovering from a stroke had been experiencing ongoing weakness in one arm and leg and decreased mental and verbal clarity. Within a few weeks after his treatment, his condition had improved 65 to 70 per cent. As a result of a car accident on Long Island, a woman suffered pain, disability and loss of balance for eighteen months. After three Maharishi Vedic Vibration Technology treatments, she was able to dispense with her cane and had largely recovered her balance.

Reports from patients are both exciting and moving. Tommie Lane, a thirty-year victim of osteoarthritis had lost the ability to close her hands fully. After three sessions, her hands not only closed, but also had regained complete flexibility and freedom from pain.

The ongoing data analysis shows that people with rheumatoid arthritis have experienced an average of 38.5 per cent relief from symptoms. One woman explained, "Rheumatoid arthritis runs in my family. The pain and swelling in my joints has been going on for two or three decades. After my consultation, the pain decreased considerably, the swelling has gone down, and it actually feels like the size of the joints is subsiding, which I never expected to happen. I'm absolutely amazed at the results."[68]

The parents of a child with attention deficit disorder reported that the treatments helped reduce their son's anger and enhanced his ability to get along with other children. A Connecticut woman found that all symptoms of colitis disappeared, while another woman found peace and relief from a lifetime of shyness.

Conditions currently being treated with the Maharishi Vedic Vibration Technology include such musculoskeletal disorders as osteo- and rheumatoid arthritis, disk problems, sciatica, heel spurs, and back pain; many other forms of pain, including headaches, neuralgia, cancer-related pain, and carpal tunnel syndrome; gastrointestinal and rectal disorders (such as anorexia, colitis, constipation, ulcers, hemorrhoids, heartburn); skin disorders (psoriasis, eczema, burning, itching); endocrine disorders; cardiovascular diseases, including hypertension and angina; mental disorders (insomnia, anxiety, depression, anger, grief, forgetfulness, etc.); Parkinson's disease; cancer; eye and ear disorders; gynecological problems; respiratory disorders; allergies; and even varicose veins.

Living Health Every Day

In a book about chronic disease, it is important not to lose sight of two of the primary purposes of this science of life, to prevent disease and promote longevity. All the approaches of Maharishi Vedic Medicine can be used to prevent disease as well as cure it. A healthy diet and daily and seasonal routine, as well as regular practice of the Transcendental Meditation technique, are crucial for maintaining health in this stressful world. Even the promise of instant healing programs does not preclude prevention. You could be cured today of migraine headaches but later develop a new set of imbalances due to wrong diet or to a strained or destructive lifestyle. What you eat and do each day is a major determinant in sustaining health and increasing longevity.

Age does not have to bring degeneration. Your daily experience of peace, vitality and fulfillment should grow along with your years, so that you can be a lighthouse for the next generation. The comprehensive wisdom of Maharishi Vedic Medicine helps you uphold wholeness in every facet of your life and the life of the entire cosmos, of which you are an intimate part.

Shifting the Focus of Medicine
from Treating Disease to Creating Health

Contemporary medicine, in its efforts to relieve symptoms and treat disease rather than patients, has lost the sense of the fundamental interconnectedness of life. Health is a state that permeates every cell, not simply isolated functions. Health describes a condition in which Nature's intelligence drives the activity of each cell without restriction, in which each cell functions perfectly within itself and in relationship to every other cell in the mind-body, in which the total individual functions with integrity within him- or herself and in relationship to every other part of the universe.

You now know that the human physiology is an expression of consciousness, the totality of Natural Law. It is structured in and administered by the immense intelligence of Nature. The fundamental cause of disease is disconnection from that unlimited organizing power, the central operating system for the human physiology and the whole cosmos. When you re-enliven this critical operating intelligence in every cell, you eliminate the fundamental cause of chronic disease and chronic pain.

Living the Full Potential of the Miracle of Life

When students are taught that the current state of affairs—the use of only 5 or 10 per cent of their potential—is normal, that life is a struggle, or that sickness and other forms of suffering are almost inevitable, those mental boundaries have physiological counterparts. The brain loses some of its ability for complete interconnectedness, and some parts of the brain are inhibited. The neuronal patterns in the brains of children take shape around the limited expectations and definitions they learn in school, at home, and from the contemporary mindset in their environment. This limited sense of life's possibilities, structured into the brain cells, sets people up to experience relatively small values of life's infinitely rich possibilities.

Health is also influenced by mental boundaries. The brain is the undisputed CEO of the nervous system and its restrictions will naturally generate physiological problems. The influence of the mind in producing disease has been clearly documented. The mind can also create health in the largest sense.

Anyone can live a miraculous life—life that not only precludes disease and suffering, but also fosters tremendous inner and outer fulfillment. This miraculous life, based on your fully realized, unlimited potential, is actually what you should consider normal. Every person can unlock the total potential of the human system and experience the perfection and organizing power of the whole cosmos. This is the goal and gift of all the therapies of Maharishi Vedic Medicine, to help each individual go beyond disease, and even beyond the need for medicine, to true health.

Information Sources on Maharishi Vedic Medicine and Related Programs

HOW TO LOCATE A PHYSICIAN
TRAINED IN MAHARISHI VEDIC MEDICINE

Contact your nearest Maharishi Vedic University, College, School, or Center, or one of the Maharishi Ayur-Veda Health Centers (see additional information later in this Appendix).

To contact Kumuda Reddy, M.D.:

    5504 Edson Lane   301-770-5690
    N. Bethesda, MD 20852
    Web site: http://www.allhealthyfamily.com

HOW TO LOCATE A TEACHER OF THE
TRANSCENDENTAL MEDITATION TECHNIQUE

Call toll-free 888-LEARN-TM (888-532-7686)
or see web site: http://www.tm.org

WHERE TO ORDER *MAHARISHI AYUR-VEDA*
TEAS AND HERBAL FORMULAS

In the United States

    Maharishi Ayur-Veda Products   800-255-8332 or
     International, Inc.   719-260-5500
    P.O. Box 49667
    Colorado Springs, CO 80949-9667
    Web site: http://www.mapi.com

In Canada

Maharishi Ayur-Veda Products Canada
P.O. Box 9402
40 Cochrane Road
Compton, Quebec J0B 1L0
Web site: http://www.all-veda.com

800-461-9685 or
819-835-5485

CENTERS OFFERING PROGRAMS IN
MAHARISHI VEDIC MEDICINE

In the United States

Maharishi Vedic Vibration Technology
Instant Relief^{6M} program
E-mail: relief@mavf.org
Web site: http://www.VedicVibration.com

800-431-9680
Fax: 603-588-2115

The Raj
Fairfield, Iowa
Web site: http://www.theraj.com

800-248-9050 or
641-472-9580

The Heavenly Mountain Clinic
Boone, North Carolina

877-890-8600

Maharishi Vedic Medical Center
Bethesda, Maryland
Web site: http://www.mvc-bethesda.org

301-770-5690
Fax: 301-770-5694

In Canada

Maharishi Ayur-Veda College
Waterville, Quebec
E-mail: cvmaha@sympatico.ca

800-575-5472 or
819-837-0772

Maharishi Ayur-Veda College
Paterson House, Ottawa, Ontario
E-mail: mavcott@istar.ca

613-565-2030
Fax: 613-565-6546

More information is available at web sites:
http://www.Maharishi-medical.com
http://www.vedic-health.com

THE *MAHARISHI VEDIC ASTROLOGY* AND *MAHARISHI YAGYA* PROGRAMS IN THE UNITED STATES AND CANADA

Maharishi Vedic Astrology program   800-888-5797
(seminars and consultations)

Maharishi Vedic Astrology and   800-483-2234
Maharishi Yagya programs   or 603-588-4235
E-mail: usayagya@Maharishi.net   Fax: 603-588-4249
Fairfield, Iowa, office   641-472-5603

More information is available at the web site:
http://www.Maharishi.org

THE *MAHARISHI STHAPATYA VEDA* PROGRAM

In response to the urgent worldwide need for people to have ideal working and living environments, Maharishi Global Construction, L.L.C. was established to offer consulting services in Maharishi Sthapatya Veda design principles to architects, designers and builders. Maharishi Global Construction is currently building Maharishi Vedic Centers and Maharishi Vedic Medical Centers around the United States.

In the United States:
Maharishi Global Construction, L.L.C.   641-472-9605
500 North Third Street, Suite 110   Fax: 641-472-9083
Fairfield, IA 52556
E-mail: reception@MGC-Vastu.com

In Canada:
Maharishi Global Construction   613-565-8525
E-mail: MGC-can@ottawa.com   Fax: 613-565-6546

More information is available at the website:
http://www.Vedahouse.com

MAHARISHI OPEN UNIVERSITY

This global university delivers the total knowledge of Natural Law via a network of eight satellites to students, working adults, and retired people in every country.

Web site: http://www.MOU.org

MAHARISHI VEDIC UNIVERSITIES, COLLEGES, SCHOOLS, AND CENTERS

Maharishi Vedic Universities, Colleges, Schools, and Centers are located in most major cities in the United States and in Canada. If you are unable to find a listing from your local telephone directory, or from directory assistance, call toll-free 888-532-7686, or see the following web site: http://www.Maharishi.org.

HEALTH EDUCATION SHORT COURSES FOR THE WHOLE POPULATION

These 16-hour courses are available at Maharishi Vedic Universities, Colleges and Schools. Full descriptions of these courses can be found at the following web site: http://www.Maharishi.org.

1. Human Physiology: Expression of Veda and the Vedic Literature
2. Good Health through Prevention
3. The Maharishi Yoga Program
4. Self-Pulse Reading Course for Prevention
5. Diet, Digestion and Nutrition
6. Maharishi Vedic Astrology Overview
7. Maharishi Vedic Architecture

DEGREE PROGRAMS

Bachelor's degree program in Maharishi Vedic Medicine and doctoral degree program in Physiology with specialization in Maharishi Vedic Medicine:

Maharishi University of Management   641-472-1150
College of Maharishi Vedic Medicine
Fairfield, IA 52557
E-mail: admissions@mum.edu
Web site: www.mum.edu/cmvm

Two-year doctor training program; A.A. degree available for beginning students (curriculum authorized by the Commission on Higher Education for the Board of Education for the State of New Mexico):

Maharishi College of Vedic Medicine   505-830-0435
2721 Arizona Street, NE   Fax: 505-830-0538
Albuquerque, NM 87110

RECOMMENDED BOOKS

Books by Maharishi Mahesh Yogi

Life Supported by Natural Law. Washington, D.C.: Age of Enlightenment Press, 1986.

Maharishi Forum of Natural Law and National Law for Doctors. India: Age of Enlightenment Publications, 1995.

Maharishi Mahesh Yogi on the Bhagavad-Gita: A New Translation and Commentary, Chapters 1-6. New York: Penguin Books, 1973.

Maharishi Vedic University: Introduction. India: Age of Enlightenment Publications, 1995.

Science of Being and Art of Living. New York: Penguin Books, 1995.

Scientific Research on Maharishi Ayur-Veda *Health Care*

Scientific Research on Maharishi's Transcendental Meditation *and* TM-Sidhi *Program: Collected Papers,* Volumes 1–6, available through Maharishi University of Management Press, Press Distribution, DB 1155, Fairfield, Iowa 52557.

Scientific Research on the Maharishi Transcendental Meditation *and* TM-Sidhi *Programs: A Brief Summary of 500 Studies.* Fairfield, Iowa: Maharishi University of Management Press, 1996.

Other Books

Nader, Tony, M.D., Ph.D. *Human Physiology: Expression of Veda and the Vedic Literature.* The Netherlands: Maharishi Vedic University Press, 1994.

Denniston, Denise. *The TM Book: How to Enjoy the Rest of Your Life.* Fairfield, Iowa: Fairfield Press, 1986.

Marcus, Jay. *The Crime Vaccine: How to End the Crime Epidemic.* Baton Rouge, Louisiana: Claitor's Publishing Division, Inc., 1996.

O'Connell, David, and Charles N. Alexander. *Self Recovery: Treating Addictions Using Transcendental Meditation and Maharishi Ayur-Veda.* New York: Haworth Press, 1994.

Roth, Robert. *Maharishi Mahesh Yogi's Transcendental Meditation.* New York: Donald I. Fine, 1994.

Sharma, Hari, M.D. *Freedom from Disease: How to Control Free Radicals, a Major Cause of Aging and Disease.* Toronto: Veda Publishing, 1993.

Wallace, R. Keith. *The Neurophysiology of Enlightenment.* Fairfield, Iowa: Maharishi International University Press, 1986.

Wallace, R. Keith. *The Physiology of Consciousness.* Fairfield, Iowa: Maharishi International University Press, 1993.

These books and others are available from
   Maharishi University of Management Press   800-831-6523
   Press Distribution DB 1155
   Fairfield, Iowa 52557
   E-mail: mumpress@mum.edu
   Web site: http://www.mum.edu/press/welcome.html

A selection of books is also available from Maharishi Ayur-Veda Products (see information above).

GLOSSARY

abhyanga Ayurvedic oil massage

agni digestive fire; also, the element of fire generally (see *mahabhuta, bhutagni, dhatu agni,* and *jatharagni*)

akasha the element of space (see *mahabhuta*)

Alochaka Pitta one of the five **subdoshas** of **Pitta**, associated with the visual system, including both outer and inner vision

ama the sticky, bad-smelling, toxic remains of undigested food that obstructs the channels in the body

ambuvaha srotas channels in the body that transport water and control water metabolism

annavaha srotas channels in the body that transport food (*anna*)

anupana ingredient added to Ayurvedic preparations to help carry them to targeted areas in the body; also used to enhance the effects or mitigate side effects

Apana Vata one of the five **subdoshas** of **Vata**, governing all downward motion in the body, particularly in the lower abdomen

apas the element of water (see *mahabhuta*)

artavavaha srotas channels that carry menstrual blood

asthi dhatu of the seven **dhatus**, **asthi** is bone tissue

asthivaha srotas channels in bone tissue

Avalambaka Kapha one of the five **subdoshas** of **Kapha**, centered in the chest, heart, and lower body; supports physical strength, the back, and stamina; regulates moisture in the lungs

Ayurveda "knowledge of the lifespan"; a major category of Vedic Literature dealing with medicine and health

bala strength or immunity

basti internal cleansing treatment for the colon

bhava "house" in Vedic astrology; twelve houses, dealing with different fields of experience, are counted from the rising sign

Bhrajaka Pitta one of the five subdoshas of **Pitta**, associated with the skin, including appearance and absorptive activity

bhutagni general term for the five types of digestive fire (***agnis***) that correspond with each of the five elements of Nature (earth, water, fire, air, space) and help to digest foods according to the presence of those elements

Bodhaka Kapha one of the five ***subdoshas*** of ***Kapha***, located in the tongue and throat; regulates secretions in the mouth as well as the sense of taste

Budha the planet Mercury

Chandra the Moon

chapati unleavened flat bread

Charaka Samhita one of the forty aspects of the Vedic Literature; the best known of the six aspects that deal explicitly with medicine and health

chhandas "the known"—one of the three fundamental divisions of consciousness (knower, knowing, and known); physiologically, corresponds with ***Kapha dosha***; mentally, corresponds with the quality known as ***tamas***

chhinna (asthma) one of the five types of asthma, "interrupted asthma"

deha prakriti one's doshic constitution at any particular point in life (see ***dosha, prakriti***)

devata "the process of knowing"—one of the three fundamental divisions of consciousness (knower, process of knowing, and known); physiologically, corresponds with ***Pitta dosha***; mentally, corresponds with the quality known as ***rajas***

Dhanu the astrological sign Sagittarius

dhatu any of the seven tissues that make up the body (see also ***dhatu agni***)

dhatu agni digestive or metabolic fire associated with each of the seven bodily tissues

dinacharya Ayurvedic daily routine

dosha any of the three fundamental operators underlying all aspects of the mind-body (see ***Vata, Pitta***, and ***Kapha***) *dravyaguna* "qualities of matter"; sophisticated science of preparing Ayurvedic herbal compounds

garshan a special massage using wool or raw silk to increase circulation in the skin

Gandharva Veda music of the ancient Vedic civilization; the eternal rhythms and melodies of Nature

gandush sesame oil gargle

ghee clarified butter, used both as a food and as a carrier to take Ayurvedic formulas to their target organs, tissues, and cells

ghrita any of several herbalized *ghees* employed for their purifying effects prior to rejuvenation treatments (see *panchakarma*)

graha "planet" in Vedic astrology

guna "quality": twenty physical qualities or gunas described by Ayurvedic texts are heavy, cold, oily, slow, stable, soft, clear, rough, gross, semisolid, light, hot, dry, rapid and acute, mobile, hard, viscous, smooth, subtle, and liquid; three mental qualities are *sattva*, *rajas*, and *tamas*

Guru the planet Jupiter

jaggary a natural form of sugar

Janma Kundali birth horoscope

jatharagni the primary digestive fire functioning in the digestive juices in the large and small intestines and the stomach, which are responsible for converting food into the nutrient plasma that nourishes all the cells and tissues throughout the body; made up of the five *bhutagnis*

Jyotish Vedic astrology

Kanya the astrological sign Virgo

Kapha one of the three mind-body operators (*doshas*); governs physical structure, including bones, muscle, and the lymphatic system, and fluid balance; primarily situated in the chest; primary qualities: heavy, oily, slow, cold, steady, solid, dull, soft, sweet, and smooth

Karka the astrological sign Cancer

kayachikitsa "therapy of fire"—the field of internal medicine used in Maharishi Rejuvenation therapy to sustain and balance the digestive fire (*agni*), including *panchakarma* and other procedures to purify and pacify the *doshas*, such as *snehana*, *swedana*, and *abhyanga*

Ketu descending lunar node—one of two points in space where the moon's path appears to cross the sun's path

kitt the waste material produced at each stage of digestion *(see also prasad)*

Kledaka Kapha one of the five *subdoshas* of *Kapha*, located in the stomach; responsible for the initial phases of digestion, especially moistening the food

kshina decrease of normal functioning of the dosha

koshta primary seat of the *doshas*, located in the intestinal tract

kshudra (asthma) simple or mild asthma

Kumbha the astrological sign Aquarius

lassi a drink made from fresh yogurt and water

maha (asthma) severe or grave asthma

mahabhuta any of the basic building blocks or elements of the material world: earth (*prithivi*), water (*apas*), fire (*tejas*), air (*vayu*) and space (*akasha*)

Maharishi Ayur-Veda health care program Ayurvedic science of health and system of medicine revived by Maharishi Mahesh Yogi

Maharishi Gandharva Veda music of the Vedic civilization, consisting of the eternal rhythms and melodies of nature, revived by His Holiness Maharishi Mahesh Yogi

Maharishi Jyotish program science of prediction—Vedic astrology—revived by Maharishi Mahesh Yogi

Maharishi Sthapatya Veda design aspect of Maharishi Vedic Science^{SM} that includes the health effects of the orientation, design, proportion, and positioning of buildings; the most ancient and supreme system of country, town, village, and home planning in accord with Natural Law

majja dhatu of the seven **dhatus**, majja includes bone marrow and the itssues of the nervous system

majjavaha srotas channels that supply the bone marrow, nerves, and brain tissue

Makara the astrological sign Capricorn

mala any of the several types of normal waste produced during formation of the **dhatus**, including urine, feces, sweat, phlegm, bile, and various other excreta

mamsa dhatu of the seven **dhatus**, mamsa is muscle tissue

mamsavaha srotas channels that nourish the muscle tissues

mandagni weak, dull digestive fire, producing heaviness in the abdomen, dullness, and breathing trouble; often a result of excess **Kapha** or eating between meals

Mangala the planet Mars

meda dhatu of the seven **dhatus**, meda is fat tissue

medavaha srotas channels that nourish the fat tissues

Meena the astrological sign Pisces

Mesha the astrological sign Aries

Mithuna the astrological sign Gemini

mutravaha srotas channels that carry urine; urinary system

nadi vigyan Ayurvedic system of pulse diagnosis

nakshatra any of the 27 divisions of a Vedic astrology chart defined by 27 fixed constellations

nasya a massage and inhalation treatment used in Maharishi Rejuvenation therapy to purify and strengthen the head, neck, shoulders, nasal passages, sinuses, and lungs; stimulates the base of the brain and produces greater clarity and balance for the mind, brain, senses, and thyroid gland

netra tarpina a treatment used in Maharishi Rejuvenation therapy in which the eyes are bathed in ghee or are exposed to herbal smoke to help cleanse impurities and relieve any kind of eye strain

Nyaya an aspect of the Vedic Literature that describes the qualities of intelligence responsible for distinguishing and deciding

ojas the most refined and nourishing product of digestion; the finest material form of consciousness

Pachaka Pitta one of the five *subdoshas* of *Pitta*, governing digestive secretions in the area of the small intestine, duodenum, and lower stomach

panchakarma "five actions"—procedures used to remove impurities from the body

pandit an expert thoroughly trained to use Vedic technologies of sound and action to restore the functioning of Natural Law through, for example, the precise performances of *yagyas*

pinda swedana a massage using cloth pouches containing herbs, rice, and milk to nourish, strengthen, and balance the joints and neuromuscular system

Pitta one of the three *doshas*; governs heat, metabolism, and energy production; primarily situated in the area around the navel; primary qualities: hot, sharp, light, acidic, slightly oily, liquid and flowing

pizzichilli a massage in which a continuous stream of warm, herbalized oil is poured over the body

prabhava the identifying characteristic of any particular herb

pragya-aparadh "mistake of the intellect"

prana breath; life force

Prana Vata one of the five *subdoshas* of *Vata*, governing movement of air, etc., in the head and chest, as well as mental clarity and sensory perception

pranavaha srotas channels that transport breath, or *prana*

pranayama neurorespiratory technique involving simple, rhythmic breathing exercises to balance, relax, and revitalize the mind-body

prasad the nutritive essence produced during digestion (*see also kitt*)

prithivi the element earth (see *mahabhuta*)

purishavaha srotas channels that carry feces; excretory system

raga musical patterns (melodies) structured according the principles of *Gandharva Veda*

Rahu ascending lunar node—one of two points in space where the moon's path appears to cross the sun's path

rajas one of the three mental qualities (*gunas*), governs the action principle, serves as the spur to action, but in an imbalanced state can give rise to agitation, anger, impulsiveness and excess (see also *sattva, tamas*)

rakta dhatu of the seven *dhatus*, rakta equates with blood

raktavaha srotas channels that transport blood and hemoglobin

Ranjaka Pitta one of the *subdoshas* of *Pitta*, governing blood chemistry and color from the liver and spleen

rasa essence or taste

rasa dhatu of the seven *dhatus*, rasa is associated with chyle, or plasma, and is the first product of digestion

rasavaha srotas channels that transport chyle to the blood and the rest of the body

rashi "sign" in Vedic astrology

rishi "knower"—one of the three fundamental divisions of consciousness (knower, knowing, and known); physiologically, it corresponds with *Vata dosha*; mentally, corresponds with the quality known as *sattva* (see also *devata, chhandas*)

ritucharya seasonal routine

Sadhaka Pitta one of the five *subdoshas* of *Pitta*, located in the heart and associated with desiring, fulfilling desires, memory, enthusiasm and energy

sama "balanced"

Sama Veda one of the four *Vedas* (*Rik, Sama, Yajur*, and *Atharva*), whose frequencies express the "flowing wakefulness" quality of Natural Law

samagni balanced digestive fire that doesn't create excessive waste, burning, gas or other digestive problems

Samana Vata one of the five *subdoshas* of *Vata*, located in the umbilical region; associated with appetite, production of digestive enzymes, and movement of food through the stomach and intestines

samhita wholeness of **rishi**, **devata**, and **chhandas**; also used in titles of many aspects of the Vedic Literature

sattva one of the three mental qualities (**gunas**); described as pure, illuminating, beneficial (see also **rajas**, **tamas**)

saumya a class of therapeutic oil used in **panchakarma** to remove physiological weakness by gently purifying one **dhatu** after another (see also **tikshana**)

Shani the planet Saturn

shirodhara a **panchakarma** treatment in which a stream of warm oil is poured back and forth in a special pattern on the forehead to settle and relax the nervous system

Shleshaka Kapha one of the five **subdoshas** of **Kapha**, responsible for the lubrication of joints

Shukra the planet Venus

shukra the subtlest of the seven **dhatus**: reproductive tissues

shukravaha srotas channels that nourish and govern the reproductive tissue

Sinha the astrological sign Leo

snehana internal purification to prepare for **panchakarma**

srota channels and microchannels within the body, such as veins, arteries, and capillaries

sthanavaha srotas channels that carry milk during lactation

Sthapatya Veda Vedic architecture; the aspect of Vedic Literature that explains the principles of orientation, design, proportion, and positioning of buildings in harmony with Natural Law; also the principles of country, town, village, and home planning in accord with Natural Law

Surya the sun

Surya Namaskara "salute to the sun"—a special sequence of asanas, or neuromuscular integration exercises

svedavaha srotas channels that carry sweat

swasthya the state of perfect health—permanent unfoldment of the deepest nature of the Self, in which state the individual is fully attuned to Natural Law

swedana a kind of steam therapy used in *panchakarma*

tamaka (asthma)   lit. "pertaining to darkness," tamaka asthma is a type of asthma identified by Ayurveda that is more severe than the more common type recognized by Western medicine

tamas one of the three mental qualties (*gunas*), generally associated with effects generated by its imbalance or excess, which produce slowness, lethargy, inertia; but when in balance, helps to stabilize growth (see also *sattva, rajas*)

tanmatra five basic forces or elements which constitute the essences of the objects of the five senses and are the precursors of the five *mahabhutas*

Tarpaka Kapha one of the five *subdoshas* of *Kapha*, located in the head and cerebrospinal fluid; responsible for nourishing and lubricating the organs of the head and for nourishing the sensory and cognitive faculties, and motor organs

tejas the element of fire, also called *agni* (see *mahabhuta*)

tikshana one of two classes of oils are used in *panchakarma* treatments which penetrate and directly enter the body; creates heat in the blood; improves circulation and purification

tikshnagni an imbalance caused by powerful or strong *agni*, in which even large amounts of food get digested too soon, producing burning in the abdomen, sour taste, thirst, heat in the body, and other problems; often caused by excess *Pitta*

Tula the astrological sign Libra

Udana Vata one of the five *subdoshas* of *Vata*, located in the throat, chest and navel

udvartana massage treatment using a paste made of ground grains; generally used to promote weight loss

urddha (asthma) "upward" asthma; an unusual variety of asthma not yet identified by Western medicine

vastu the correct relationship between a building site and the environment

Vata the "king" of the three mind-body operators *doshas*, because it leads *Pitta* and *Kapha* in responding to internal and external factors; governs motion of all kinds—mental, physical, emotional— from its primary seat in the colon

vayu the element of air (see *mahabhuta*)

Veda "knowledge"—total knowledge and structure of Natural Law expressed in unmanifest frequencies of sound that precede and produce the physical manifestation of the universe

vikriti a state of imbalance in the doshas characterized by an excess of one or more *doshas*

vipaka the post-digestive effect or aftertaste of an herb

virechana laxative therapy used in *panchakarma*

virya potency (of an herb)

vriddhi increase or aggravation of one or another *dosha*

Vrishabha the astrological sign Taurus

Vrishchika the astrological sign Scorpio

vishmagni erratic *agni* that fluctuates from meal to meal, causing gas, cramping, constipation, and other obstructions to normal elimination; often linked to *Vata* aggravation.

Vyana Vata one of the five *subdoshas* of *Vata*; governs circulation of blood, lymph, and sweat, as well as nerve impulses promoting, for example, extension and contraction of muscles

vyavai vikasi a healing process that eradicates blockages, dispels pain and heaviness, and inhibits the effects of pollutants to which the body is exposed, through the mechanism of herbalized oil massage

Yoga asanas neuromuscular integration exercises

Yoga Sutras one of the forty branches of Vedic Literature, which structures the brain's association fibers in the cerebral cortex; and noted for its unifying quality

INDEX

Page numbers with definitions are in italics.

NOTES

1. Maharishi Mahesh Yogi, *Maharishi Forum of Natural Law and National Law for Doctors* (India: Age of Enlightenment Publications, 1955), p. 44.

2. C. Hoffman, D. Rice, and H.Y. Sung, "Persons with Chronic Conditions: Their Prevalence and Costs," *JAMA*, vol. 276, no. 18, (Nov. 13, 1996), pp. 1473–1479.

3. Ibid.

4. *JAMA*, vol. 272 (1994), pp. 1851–1857.

5. See Maharishi Vedic Approach to Health web site, http://www.vedic-health.com/hazards/medical hazards, p. 3.

6. *Time*, Sept. 29, 1997. Article content drawn from *JAMA*, the Centers for Disease Control, and the Archives of General Psychiatry.

7. Maharishi Mahesh Yogi, *Maharishi Forum of Natural Law and National Law for Doctors* (India: Age of Enlightenment Publications, 1995), p. 53.

8. Maharishi Mahesh Yogi, *Maharishi Forum of Natural Law and National Law for Doctors* (India: Age of Enlightenment Publications, 1995), p. 64.

9. *Charaka Samhita*, Sharirasthana 4:13

10. Maharishi Mahesh Yogi, *Maharishi Forum of Natural Law and National Law for Doctors* (India: Age of Enlightenment Publications, 1995), p. 219.

11. Maharishi Mahesh Yogi, *Maharishi Forum of Natural Law and National Law for Doctors* (India: Age of Enlightenment Publications, 1995), p. 53.

12. *Charaka Samhita*, Sutrasthana 28:39–40.

13. *Charaka Samhita*, Sutrasthana 1:54–55.

14. Maharishi Mahesh Yogi, *Maharishi Forum of Natural Law and National Law for Doctors*, (India: Age of Enlightenment Publications, 1995), p. 35

15. *Charaka Samhita*, Sutrashtana 5:45.

16. *Charaka Samhita*, Sutrasthana 17:62.

17. *Charaka Samhita*, Sutrasthana 28: 31–32.

18. *Charaka Samhita*, Sutrasthana 1:54.

19. *Charaka Samhita*, Chikitsasthana 15:3–5.

20. *Charaka Samhita*, Sutrasthana 27:342.

21. *Charaka Samhita*, Vimanasthana 5:23.

22. *Charaka Samhita*, Vimanasthana 5:6.

23. *Charaka Samhita*, Vimanasthana 5:10–22.

24 *Charaka Samhita*, Sutrasthana 20:9–10.
25 *Charaka Samhita*, Chikitsa 28:58–60.
26 Maharishi Mahesh Yogi, *Maharishi Forum of Natural Law and National Law for Doctors* (India: Age of Enlightenment Publications, 1995), p. 35.
27 James W. Long, M.D., *The Essential Guide to Chronic Illness* (New York: Harper Collins, 1997), pp. 371–373.
28 See Maharishi Vedic Approach to Health web site, http://www.vedic-health.com/arthritis/arthritishazards.html
29 James W. Long, M.D., *The Essential Guide to Chronic Illness* (New York: Harper Collins, 1997), p. 71.
30 Nagendra Nath Sen Gupta, *The Ayurvedic System of Medicine* (New Delhi: Logos Press, 1919).
31 Maharishi Mahesh Yogi, *Maharishi Forum of Natural Law and National Law for Doctors* (India: Age of Enlightenment Publications, 1995), p. 53.
32 Maharishi Mahesh Yogi, *Maharishi Forum of Natural Law and National Law for Doctors* (India: Age of Enlightenment Publications, 1995), p. 59.
33 *Charaka Samhita*, Vimanasthana 8:94.
34 Eric J. Cassell, M.D., *The Healer's Art: A New Approach to the Doctor-Patient Relationship* (New York: J. B. Lippencott Company, 1976), p. 99.
35 *Perfect Health and Immortality: Reversing the Aging Process through the Transcendental Meditation and TM-Sidhi Program* (Fairfield, Iowa: Maharishi International University Press, 1980), p. 4.
36 Maharishi Mahesh Yogi, *Vedic Knowledge for Everyone* (Holland: Maharishi Vedic University Press, 1994), p. 288.
37 *Charaka Samhita*, Sutrasthana 1:6–23.
38 *Charaka Samhita*, Sutrasthana 27:349–350.
39 *Charaka Samhita*, Sutrasthana 28:348.
40 Hari M. Sharma, M.D., *Indian Journal of Clinical Practice*, vol. 1, no. 2 (July 1990).
41 *Charaka Samhita*, Chikitsasthana 5:136.
42 *Charaka Samhita*, Chikitsasthana 1:7–8.
43 *Charaka Samhita*, Sutrasthana 1:68–73.
44 V. Sundaram, M.D., A.N. Hanna, Ph.D., G.P. Lubow, M.D., L. Koneru, M.D., J.M. Falko, M.D., and H.M. Sharma, MD, FRCPC, "Effect of Herbal Mixtrues MAK-4 and MAK-5 on Susceptibility of Human LDL to Oxidation," *American Journal of the Medical Sciences*, vol. 314, no. 5 (1997), pp. 303–310.
45 H.M. Sharma, C. Dwivedi, B.C. Satter, K.P. Gudehithlu, H. Abou-Issa,

W. Malarkey, and G.A. Tejwani, "Antineoplastic Properties of Maharishi-4 [MAK-4] Against DMVA-Induced Mammary Tumors in Rats," *Pharmacology, Biochemistry and Behavior*, vol. 34 (1990), pp. 767–773.

[46] Ibid.

[47] *Charaka Samhita*, Sutrasthana 5:85–89.

[48] Maharishi Mahesh Yogi, *Maharishi Forum of Natural Law and National Law for Doctors* (India: Age of Enlightenment Publications, 1995), p. 50.

[49] M.M. Stevens, J. Campbell, and D.E. Smith, "Reduction in Bacterial Colony Types Associated with Sesame Oil Mouthrinse." Abstract presented at the International Symposium on Dental Hygiene, Ottawa, Canada, June 28, 1989.

[50] *Charaka Samhita*, Sutrasthana 5:103–104.

[51] *Charaka Samhita*, Sutrasthana 5:78–80.

[52] *Charaka Samhita*, Sutrasthana 7:32.

[53] *Charaka Samhita*, Sutrasthana 6:3.

[54] *Charaka Samhita*, Sutrasthana 6:50.

[55] Maharishi Mahesh Yogi, *Maharishi Forum of Natural Law and National Law for Doctors* (India: Age of Enlightenment Publications, 1995), pp. 306–307.

[56] *Charaka Samhita*, Sutrasthana 16:20–21.

[57] Maharishi Mahesh Yogi, *Maharishi Forum of Natural Law and National Law for Doctors* (India: Age of Enlightenment Publications, 1995), p. 190.

[58] D.C. MacClelland, "Music in the Operating Room," *AORN Journal*, vol. 29, no. 2 (1979), pp. 252–260.

[59] J.D. Cook, "Music as an Intervention in the Oncology Setting," *Cancer Nursing*, vol. 9, no. 1 (1986), pp. 23–28.

[60] H.M. Sharma, E.M. Kauffman, and R.E. Stephens, "Effect of Different Sounds on Growth of Human Cancer Cell Lines in Vitro," *Alternative Therapies in Clinical Practice*, vol. 3, no. 4 (1996), pp. 25–32.

[61] *Designs According to Maharishi Sthapatya Veda* (Fairfield, Iowa: Maharishi Global Construction, L.L.C., 1997).

[62] Maharishi Mahesh Yogi, *Maharishi Forum of Natural Law and National Law for Doctors* (India: Age of Enlightenment Publications, 1995), p. 54.

[63] Maharishi Mahesh Yogi, *Maharishi Forum of Natural Law and National Law for Doctors* (India: Age of Enlightenment Publications, 1995), p. 313.

[64] Andrea's and Sonia's accounts excerpted with permission from "En-

couraging Self-Repair: New Centers for Chronic Diseases Offer Hope for Previously Untreatable Problems," by Eva Herriott, *The Iowa Source*, vol. 14, no. 10 (December 1997), p. F-6. For complete case histories, see T. Nader, M.D., Ph.D.; S. Rothenberg, M.D.; R. Averbach, M.D.; B. Charles, M.D.; J.Z. Fields, M.D.; R. Schneider, M.D.; "Improvements in Chronic Disease with a Comprehensive Natural Medicine Approach: A Review and Case Studies," *Behavioral Medicine*, vol. 26 (2000) pp. 34–46.

[65] Maharishi Mahesh Yogi, *Maharishi Forum of Natural Law and National Law for Doctors* (India: Age of Enlightenment Publications, 1995), p. 243.

[66] Tony Nader, M.D., Ph.D., *Human Physiology—Expression of Veda and the Vedic Literature* (Netherlands: Maharishi Vedic University, 1995).

[67] Arenander, Alarik, Ph.D., "Total Brain Development" in *Enlightenment*, vol. 2, no. 1 (Antrim, NH: Maharishi Vedic Education Development Corporation, March, 1999), p. 14.

[68] Lara L. Reutlinger-Haight, "Vedic Sounds Ease Arthritic Pain," in *Relief*, vol. 1, no. 1 (Antrim, NH: Maharishi Vedic Foundation, 1999), p. 10.